HOSPITAL OF HORROR

At first, doctors at the Veterans Hospital in Ann Arbor, Michigan, tried to ascribe the puzzling deaths by sudden respiratory failure to natural causes. But as the grim toll mounted, a shocking suspicion grew inescapable. Someone was stalking the hospital, hypodermic in hand, injecting patients with a deadly drug that was virtually impossible to detect.

Now, for the first time, we have the whole story of this macabre case of menace and mystery: the hideous deaths themselves; the potent drug with its awesome powers; the enthralling medical and police detective work, including the use of a New York hypnotist; the two nurses charged with the crime; and the terrifying questions that remain even now.

Here, from an award-winning reporter, is a tale that overshadows any fiction in its fearsome fascination and riveting revelation.

**Unable to find
your favorite Popular Library books?**

If you are unable to locate a book published by Popular Library, or, if you wish to see a list of all available Popular Library titles, write for our FREE catalog to:

Popular Library
Reader Service Department
P.O. Box 5755
Terre Haute, Indiana 47805

(Please enclose 25¢ to help pay for postage and handling)

THE MYSTERIOUS DEATHS AT ANN ARBOR

by Robert K. Wilcox

POPULAR LIBRARY • NEW YORK

All POPULAR LIBRARY books are carefully selected by the POPULAR LIBRARY Editorial Board and represent titles by the world's greatest authors.

POPULAR LIBRARY EDITION

May, 1977

Copyright © 1977 by Robert K. Wilcox

ISBN: 0-445-04030-0

PRINTED IN THE UNITED STATES OF AMERICA

All Rights Reserved

Acknowledgments

I would like to thank Eric C. Hodeen, M. D., for his reading of the first ten chapters for possible medical errors. I would also like to thank Marge Keasler for her editing of the manuscript before it went to the publisher, and Elinor Smith, director of Elinor Smith Executive Secretaries, Inc. Coral Gables, Fla. I am grateful to both for their help. Finally, I would like to thank those doctors, official investigators, and Ann Arbor VA employees who spoke candidly to me about things in spite of the overall climate of secrecy, suspicion, and hostility at the hospital. I cannot name them because I promised I wouldn't. But I am grateful for their decency.

R. K. W.

Chapter 1

The evening was cool and still. Outside the Ann Arbor, Michigan, Veterans Administration Hospital the calm was broken only by the lights and noise of passing cars. The hospital loomed dark and menacing. Clumped on a land triangle between two outskirt city roads, its massive red brick buildings, ten stories high in places, appeared black—giant, chunky boxes intersecting each other with rows of tiny lighted windows dotting their façades. A huge smokestack jutted skyward from its dense interior.

It was a night in late July 1975, and something terrible was about to happen in the government institution.

Inside, the dimly lit corridors were mostly deserted. Visiting hours had ended and the staff was a skeleton of its daylight size. There had been complaints about the understaffing. The work load was too great and crisis-handling might be impaired. But the money to put more people on simply was not available. The lighted security office across from the first-floor elevators appeared empty. Guards were off checking doors, or on some other duty.

On the third floor the intensive care unit (ICU) was

full. Several nurses attended patients, mostly older men. One sat at the nurse's station. There were approximately eleven patients—the majority in beds set around an open ward. Some were in private glass-enclosed rooms. Tubes sprouted from their bodies. Intravenous bags (IVs) dripped fluids into their veins. The majority were unconscious. All were heavily drugged. They lay ashen and naked, except for loosely draped hospital gowns, and occasionally one jerked in uncontrollable spasm. An eerie atmosphere permeated the unit. Constant artificial light obliterated the normal distinctions between night and day, blue-green lines blipped across luminous monitors, and mechanical life-support machines hummed, hissed and wheezed incessantly in the background.

Totally dependent, the patients were at the mercy of their attendants.

At one of the beds, a figure in white, it is now believed, walked over to stand beside a dozing eighty-eight-year-old man, unnoticed. Hospital personnel were constantly at the bedsides of patients—especially in the ICU. Even if the person's presence had been noticed it most probably would have been forgotten; it was perfectly normal for a nurse, aide or doctor to have been there.

In the person's hand was a small syringe, partially concealed, but not actively hidden. It was also commonplace for syringes to be in the hands of hospital personnel, especially in the ICU. The syringe's small chamber contained a clear liquid generically called pancuronium, but more commonly known in the hospital by its trade name, Pavulon, a manufacturer's term. The person may have stared at the old man a moment before squeezing the syringe until a drop formed at its tip.

Pavulon is synthetic curare, a poison derived from

special tropical plants and used, for instance, by South American jungle Indians on the tips of darts shot to kill game. In a hospital, however, it is a surgical and recovery aid. It is a paralyzer. Injected into the human body, as it sometimes is under controlled conditions, it disrupts the delicate communication between nerves and the brain-message receptors on certain muscles, such as the diaphragm, which controls breathing. The result is that once the drug has taken hold—and that occurs quite rapidly, especially with Pavulon, which is one of the most powerful muscle relaxers—many of the muscles, including the diaphragm, cease to function. Tracheal tubes then, for instance, can be easily inserted during an operation.

Patients are never given muscle relaxers, in surgery or elsewhere, unless they are connected to a mechanical respirator which can then do their breathing for them. But the patient lying prone and oblivious in front of the person was not on a respirator.

Quickly, and with experienced precision, the figure moved in close, covering his or her actions with its body, and inserted the needle's tip into a rubber coupling device at the top of one of the patient's many IV tubes. A small bolus of clear fluid entered the line and began a slow descent to the patient's arm, propelled by each drop of IV fluid above it. Probably dropping the syringe into a pocket, the person turned away from the old man and meshed into the maze of equipment and several attendants on the floor. The old man slept on.

At the nurse's station, which has a view of practically everything in the unit, someone is charged with monitoring all the patients. Shortly after the figure in white left the bedside someone noticed that the labored breathing of the old man had abruptly halted. "Respiratory arrest," as a sudden breathing stoppage is called, is a crisis situation. It is similar to "cardiac arrest," where the heartbeat has suddenly stopped. And whoever noticed the old man immediately gave the alarm. Attendants rushed to the bedside. A button was pushed which instantly flashed red wall lights with "7" on them throughout the hospital. The light is a signal that a "Code 7"—a medical emergency—has been called, and everyone available drops what he or she is doing and runs to offer help.

Doctors are summoned on beepers carried in their pockets.

Those first at the scene make sure the victim's airway is clear and then clasp what is called an "ambu" bag over his mouth and nose. It is a bladder-like device and the rescuers are able to begin pumping air into the victim's lungs by squeezing and releasing it. In a short time—whenever the equipment is available, and it should be close by in the ICU—an "intubation" begins.

A curved, flexible tube is inserted down the victim's throat. The tube is hooked up to a mechanical respirator and the machine switched on to take over. Shortly, a steady wheeze about every four seconds indicates the respirator is doing its job. The doctors now have time—if they haven't done so already—to check the patient for any complications that may have developed. Medications may be necessary. Luckily, in this case, they quickly concluded, no other damage had occurred. The momentary loss of oxygen to the brain had not resulted in any complication. The respiratory arrest had not had time to build into a cardiac arrest.

When breathing stops, heart stoppage is soon to follow. Conversely cardiac arrest will eventually cause respiratory arrest. The two go hand in hand.

The patient was now awake. He was stabilized. His mouth bulged with the intubation tube. He could not talk, but his eyes were wide and darting. He didn't know what had happened, but it was obvious that he was very frightened. He clutched the sheet beneath him and sweat beaded on his forehead despite the fact that it was cool in the ICU. Later he would talk about having had a terrible dream. Nightmares sometimes accompany body trauma. Had he been awake when he received the injection, the following is what he might have experienced:

About forty-five seconds to two minutes after the Pavulon had entered his bloodstream he would have begun to feel a tingling—perhaps even a stinging—all over. Rapidly his extremities would have started to falter. He might have made a move toward his head because something strange was happening in his upper body. It suddenly would have become clear that he was rapidly losing the ability to breath.

But his arms would have quickly fallen to his sides. He most probably would not have had time to call out. Then his eyelids would have fallen shut with horrible finality. His immobility would have been complete. He would not have been able to lift even a little finger to help himself. Wanting desperately to cry out for help, he would not even have been able to make his eyeballs move beneath the closed lids.

Every skeletal muscle would have been rendered flaccid, as pliable and unresponsive as a slab of meat in a butcher's hand. But there would have been no loss of feeling. His brain would have continued to function for a time, receiving messages from the nerves that record pain. Every needle injected into him, every fist smashed into his chest—as is often done in resuscitations—every wrenching of the neck to open the airway for reception of the intubation tube would have been felt.

And voices would have been heard. As, from the darkness all around him, the nurses and doctors might have commanded him to breathe, or maybe shouted among themselves that he seemed dead and they may as well relax their frantic efforts to revive him, he might have desperately wanted to scream back, "Save me!" But he couldn't have uttered a word. All he could have done was listen—and pray.

Moreover, he would have been fully cognizant of the horrible feeling of suffocation slowly creeping up within him. Like a man held under water, he would have been bursting for air. But it might have been two or three minutes before relief came. That relief, however, would have been as dreaded, perhaps more so, as the suffocation.

The most terrifying aspect of the injection he had received would have soon become clear—impending death. A sinister blackness would have begun to engulf him as he realized he was suffocating, and he would have been powerless to do anything about it. Like a man buried alive, he would have been forced to lie immobile, his heart pounding in his brain (for although the skeletal muscles are affected, the heart is not), until unconsciousness—the dreaded unconsciousness—slowly took him away. Death would have followed shortly thereafter.

He would not even have had the psychological relief of being able to scream and writhe until it was done.

But the old man, luckily, probably had not experienced any of this—at least not consciously. And the code 7 team, most likely, was totally ignorant of what might have been going on. Had they been studying the incidence of respiratory arrest at the hospital they might have had an inkling. The number of such arrests had, by mid-July, already passed the normal monthly rate of eight and was many times that rate now. Also, the number of monthly deaths at the hospital had been rising steadily since March, and July—the current month—was breaking all records. There would be twenty-eight deaths recorded by July's end, the highest in any month in the entire year and thirteen above the monthly average of fifteen recorded in the first six months of 1975.

But the statistics had not yet been compiled—at least not for distribution. Most in the ICU that night were aware that there had been a lot of arrests lately. But few, if any, had access to daily compilations. And summer is traditionally a bad time in hospitals anyway. In addition, the old man was very sick. He had had a serious operation and complications. It was not unexpected that he would have problems. That was the reason he was in the ICU. True, he had seemed to be coming along fine. But the incidence of arrest in elderly patients is far greater than in young ones. And sick old patients are primary candidates for both cardiac and respiratory arrest.

The old man was now stabilized and doing reasonably well. The intubation had been a success. The team began to break up. Its members moved back to the jobs they had been doing before the arrest was called.

None of them suspected.

Outside the ICU, the corridors seemed especially deserted. Those few who might have been walking around in them were probably involved in the Code 7. But at least one figure might have been visible, moving quietly in the dim light. It was a short distance to the elevator and then only one floor to the urology-orthopedic ward, where patients with urinary tract and bone problems were kept. No matter what their problems, these patients were not as sick as those in the ICU. Consequently, even without a Code 7 in progress, there would be fewer attendants there.

At this particular moment, it is believed, only one was in sight. She was at the nurse's station, her eyes probably looking down, her mind concentrating on something she was doing. In front of her was a long, dark hall. The light was so dim down the hall that the farthest room entrances could barely be made out. Two other dark halls ran off the sides of the station.

Intent on what she was doing, the nurse never would have seen the figure go silently by her.

In his room, a sixty-one-year-old patient prepared to sleep. IVs dripped into his body. He, too, recently had had an operation. His bladder had been removed; cancerous tumors had been found in it. But he'd been reassured that there was a good chance the problem was licked. Despite his discomfort, he was resting.

As he began to close his eyes, probably foggy with medicine, he became aware that someone was standing near him. He could make out a figure through the maze of IVs hanging at his bedside, but he was not too concerned. Frequently people were tampering with his medications—adjusting the drip rate or changing one of the container bags. He was tired and wanted only to close his eyes.

Suddenly, he opened them again. Something was happening, he realized. He didn't know what, but he didn't like it. He started to rise. Then, on impulse, a cry issued from his lips: "Hey, nurse!" It was a cry for help. But he was only able to shout once. Almost as soon as the air had been expelled from his mouth he dropped back hard to his pillow. Out of the corner of his eye he saw the figure standing there, then run out. After that everything seemed to go black. He heard voices for a while, but he could see nothing.

Someone, perhaps the nurse at the station at the front of the hall, heard his cry, for attendants were at his bedside within moments—a male and a female nurse. The patient was blue by the time they got there, and a Code 7 was promptly flashed. Manual resuscitation was performed until a doctor arrived and began the more complicated procedures. Later the patient would recall: "All of a sudden I began losing my breath. Then I was paralyzed. I couldn't move a leg or foot or arm or nothin'. But I could hear voices talkin'."

But mostly his mind was a blank about what had happened.

Oftentimes the mind erases what is deemed too terrible to recall.

It was the second respiratory arrest that night, and although the doctors thought it odd that this patient, many days post-op and seemingly on his way to a solid recovery, would have had a sudden breathing failure, they decided that perhaps, as occasionally happens, a complication had developed of which they had not been aware. Perhaps a blood clot had formed during surgery, for instance, and traveled to the lung, thereby causing the malfunction. It was certainly possible.

In reality, the doctors that night had no explanation for the arrest. But that in itself was not rare. Sometimes the unexplainable things that happen in hospitals—and there are many—are simply chalked up to an elusive unknown. No one knows everything, nor can he be expected to.

The patient was taken to the ICU, where he was later stabilized.

Again, no one appeared to suspect anything sinister.

Above, on the fifth floor, a third patient, seventy-four, a double amputee, could have heard the commotion but would have paid little attention: he was too sick. A diabetic and an alcoholic, he had entered the hospital for tests. But something unexpected had gone wrong inside him and his temperature was now very high. He might have been moaning with pain; he had been receiving pain-killers and their effects might have worn off. Sleep and pain had been coming to him alternately in waves. He had just awakened, it can be speculated, for the third time in an hour.

He shifted, trying to get another position in bed, and suddenly, his vision impaired with fever, he became aware of the presence of another person in the room. He squinted but was unable to focus. All he could have seen was a figure holding what looked like a syringe, standing there before him. For an instant he might have been apprehensive, his eyebrows hunched with concern. But then the pain would have come rushing back. His eyes probably dropped to the syringe and he might have begged: "Quick, quick, give it to me."

He would have turned away, waiting for what he believed to be a pain-killer. The syringe's needle entered an IV line.

Shortly, a ringing sound would have started in the amputee's ears—the kind of sound one hears in absolute silence. Something strange and ominous was occurring, he would have realized. Suddenly he would have been aware of a deadening in his throat. He may have tried to raise his hands but they would have dropped. His body would have gone limp. There would have been an audible gasp as the last bit of air left his lungs. His body would then have been totally lifeless. But a queer look on his face, ghostly in what little light came in from the corridor, might have indicated that he was still alive—only unable to breathe: a conscious man inside a functionless body.

If one had been able to get inside his brain at that moment there would have been a screaming sense of helplessness and the dull sound of two heels padding rhythmically along the corridor outside. It's quite possible that an attendant might have been walking to the nurse's station, unaware that the slightly ajar door he was passing opened to a paralyzed man who was praying he would enter and help.

But no help came. The third victim that night wasn't found until it was too late, his body cold and growing stiff.

Another Code 7 was called, but respondents saw it was too late when they arrived. It had been an exhausting evening, and they probably slumped at the sight. Most doctors and nurses hate to lose patients' lives no matter what the circumstances. Not only are they professionally involved, but they often have come to know the patients personally. They would have felt particularly bad this time because they didn't even have a chance to try to prevent the death.

Down in the morgue, they doubtless discussed what might have happened. The patient was relatively old. He had several chronic problems. The diabetes had already taken his legs. His will to live was not strong. It was only a matter of time before his problems were expected to finish him. The internal infection he was lately suffering from had turned septic, meaning it had broken out of confinement and had filled his bloodstream with deadly bacteria. Fierce chills and fever must have accompanied his death. His pelvis was inflamed. He had been a kidney patient for years, and the infection inside had done particular damage there.

Again, the arrest was ascribed to natural causes—at least to those ailments that were naturally present. The death certificate was filled out without the slightest hint that anything out of the ordinary might have occurred. Even the fact that the three Code 7s were close together in time and place caused no comment, though three attacks at the same time were abnormal. The normal rate of arrests at the hospital had been barely two per week. But lately there had been many multiple Code 7s—especially on the night shift.

Subconsciously the staff was beginning to expect them.

"You'd think we had a phantom arrester," one doctor joked to an orderly. Neither, as they walked away, realized the truth in what he said.

Chapter 2

The preceding is based on fact. It is a recounting of events which federal investigators believe took place in those dark days of late July. What has deliberately been left vague are events not yet proven. The killer (or killers), for instance, has not yet been tried. His, or her (or their), actions can only be speculated upon—like missing pieces of a jigsaw puzzle. But the speculation is based on known facts about the killer's method.

Two of the victims depicted—the cancer patient and the double amputee—did suffer mysterious arrests, believed to be attacks with Pavulon, and in the manner described. The cancer victim's name is Richard Neely, an Indiana factory worker; the amputee, John Herman, a retired Michigan machinist. The night they are believed to have been attacked was July 30, on which, as described, there were three fast-breaking emergency codes at the hospital. What happened to Neely is based on his own recollections. Since Herman was found dead, however, no one will ever really know what happened to him. The depiction presented, based on hospital records and sources, and interviews with his family, represents one of the darkest possibilities.

It does not appear that the old man in the ICU, Charles Gasmire, also a Michigan man and a former insurance salesman, suffered the arrest on the date described. But because the arrest occurred in the ICU (and most of the attacks during that fateful period took place in the ICU), including it seems representative. It is a way to give an accurate picture of what is believed by investigators to have been going on at the hospital in late July—the time when hospital authorities first began to realize something was wrong.

But the story of the Ann Arbor Veterans Administration Hospital murders, which, when the final chapter is written, might include as many as fifteen dead victims and many more who were attacked, actually began earlier in the summer, when new doctors and medical students came to the hospital eager to begin what they thought at that time would be the happy and relatively uneventful start of new careers and learning experiences.

The Ann Arbor Veterans Administration Hospital is probably average size for a VA hospital. Opened in 1953, in response to the Korean War, it has an approximate 460-bed capacity, although the average number of patients is around 300. Full capacity would pack patients in like sardines. A distinction is that it is one of the VA hospitals in the country with a liaison with a university. The University of Michigan is located in Ann Arbor and under a special program worked out, hopefully to give better patient care, the UM medical school sends groups of med students and post-graduate residents to the VA to work, train and learn under the VA's small permanent staff.

July 1, 1975, was one of the major turnover dates in the program. An academic year had just ended. Approximately seventy new med students and residents began coming to the VA at that time. And, at first, some people thought this might be the reason for the rising number of codes.

The hospital functions in pyramid style. At the base are med students and interns, doctors (also called first-year residents) who have recently graduated and are serving required time in various specialties. These doctors and student doctors are integrated into the hospital's medical divisions, including internal medicine, dermatology, allergy, general surgery, urology, ophthalmology, otolaryngology, orthopedic surgery, psychiatry, neurology, anesthesiology, thoracic surgery and dentistry. Higher-level residents supervise them. Supervising all the young doctors and doctor trainees are older, more experienced VA permanent staff members, perhaps numbering forty doctors.

Each specialty in the hospital has a permanent staff head. The two largest specialties, called "services," are internal medicine and surgery, under which many of the subspecialties come. All medical personnel—med students, residents and permanent staff members—are under a chief of staff, a doctor appointed by the UM who maintains close contact with the university's medical school. The chief of staff reports only to the hospital's chief administrator, a layman who relies on the doctors to tell him what medically is going on, and who devotes his time to the business of running the hospital.

Under the teaching program, the permanent staff that summer as always, had little patient contact. Day-to-day patient care was left mostly to the young doctors; they were the ones there to learn. Only in special cases would the permanent staff step in and administer care themselves. Theirs was largely a background role—running the program, making important decisions, watching that everything went properly.

On the one hand, the hospital proudly boasted that the program allowed it to maintain a high ratio of doctors to patients. There were always many doctors around, certainly more than in most VA hospitals. And since the doctors were from the university and their superiors were university-connected—every permanent staff member had a teaching post at the UM—the quality of care was higher than average. But critics—mostly patients' families who had a grievance with the hospital—charged that patients were guinea pigs.

The patients themselves were largely elderly and indigent, and several VA doctors reported a high incidence of alcoholism. The majority had served in World War II, although there were World War I, Korean and Vietnam veterans. At one point during the investigation, the hospital's chief of staff was quoted as saying 85 per cent of the patients were non-paying. While the doctors and med students were mostly polished, middle and upper middle class with a conspicuous number from eastern U.S. cities like New York, the patients were largely from the lower economic groups: farmers, factory workers, small-town men who spent long hours standing at assembly lines in Detroit auto plants or working small plots of land.

But the differences between the two groups were seldom of any importance to the young doctors, who for the most part seemed instilled with a high degree of professional competence and regard for patients. They seemed bright, conscientious and eager, and most patients probably felt lucky to be in the Ann Arbor VA that summer.

Although hospital officials did not begin to sense something might be wrong at the VA until late July, it appears that danger signals were surfacing before that time.

For instance, the number of respiratory arrests or

Code 7s at the hospital appears to have exceeded the normal monthly rate of eight, or two per week, by as early as mid-July. Available records—and such things are scarce because hospital officials refuse to release to outsiders any detailed information about the suspected murders—indicate that as many as fifteen respiratory arrests had been recorded by July 18, twice the normal monthly rate.

Similarly, the number of deaths at the hospital was rising noticeably at the same time. By the nineteenth, the number of deaths had already exceeded the first half of 1975's monthly average of approximately fifteen deaths per month. Equally ominous was the fact that by the same date the hospital had experienced three different days in which three or more patients had died: the fifth, on which four had died; the tenth, on which three had died; and the nineteenth, on which three had died.

The hospital's normal daily death rate at that time was approximately one death every other day.

But statistics are seldom of any use until after the fact—at least in a case like this. Some of the young doctors, the ones having most of the patient contact, recall being aware of a heightened number of respiratory arrests during those early days, but little more. Also, their lack of experience kept them in the dark about the meaning of the development. "I knew we were having a lot of arrests," says one, "but as far as I knew it wasn't out of the ordinary. I'd never worked in the VA before. I didn't know what the normal arrest rate was."

In late July both the arrest and death rates took sharp turns upward. From the twenty-fifth of July to the thirty-first there were approximately twelve respiratory arrests at the hospital. Instead of having two arrests per week, which was average, the hospital was having two per day. The sudden increase jumped the total number of arrests to above thirty by the thirty-first, an average of nearly one per day throughout the month, or nearly four times the normal monthly average. In the nine days between July 23 and 31, there were, in addition, twelve deaths at the hospital, three times the average number of deaths for a similar period in previous months.

Further, beginning in late July, the arrests began coming in clusters. Normally arrests are separated in both time and place. But beginning around the twenty-sixth, the Code 7s began to come in bunches. On the twenty-sixth, there were two in the ICU, both around noon. On the twenty-seventh and twenty-eighth, there were four more, at least three of which are known to have taken place in the ICU. On the twenty-ninth, there were three, possibly four, in the ICU—all around 10:30 P.M. And on the thirtieth, as described in Chapter 1, there were three—the cancer patient and amputee among them.

"We'd no sooner rush to one patient then the nurses would call us to another," recalls one doctor about this period.

Four veterans died on the twenty-fifth and three on the thirty-first, bringing the total number of deaths for July to twenty-eight by the month's end—the highest number in any month for at least the past two years and thirteen above the average for any 1975 month previous to it.

Clearly something was wrong.

But few people in the hospital seem to have been fully cognizant of what was happening in late July. One reason may have been that almost all the arrests at that time and in the days to come were occurring at night. While the hospital was at full staff in the daytime, only a fraction was on at night—perhaps thirty persons altogether (although, counting late-working residents, as many as fifty might be in the hospital—as opposed to hundreds during the day. All the hospital's supervisors were home. And because of rotation, the few doctors who alternately worked the night shift were seldom in a position to see any continuing trends.

During the nights, only two doctors were officially on duty at the hospital—one from the medical service and one from the surgical service, called MOD (medical officer of the day) and SOD (surgical officer of the day). The two doctors were always young residents. Seldom, if ever, would any one of them work two days in a row. Usually it was one night every week. Few, if any, ever had a chance to see more than four or five nights of arrests per month.

Even if an MOD or SOD did experience an abnormal number of arrests or deaths on his periodic nights, he believed it to be just a freak or isolated occurrence. Not being an administrator, he would not be looking at day-to-day statistics. And with a heavy work load, seldom would he have a chance to compare experiences with other residents.

A resident from Miami, Florida, who served during the period relates:

"Once we had this strange arrest—a patient who shouldn't have had a respiratory failure. He wasn't my patient, but, being there, I put the question to myself, why is this patient having an arrest? Then I saw that he was receiving blood. It is known that blood transfusions can lead to a certain reaction called anaphylaxis and you stop breathing. I discussed this with the surgeon who was responsible and I left.

"I never heard any more about it. Then it turns out that this guy subsequently becomes one of the primary suspect cases. But at the time it never occurred to me he was being poisoned. My natural reaction had been to think what medical thing was going on. The only thing that came to mind was that this guy was receiving a transfusion and it fit.

"If I had been taking care of that patient full time I probably would have found out that the transfusion was not the cause. But I wasn't. I left. I figured the other doctor should know. But because he, too, isn't talking with the others he probably thinks it was an isolated case and forgets about it. The fact that it was strange is forgotten. He doesn't know that three other guys have had the same experience."

However, the mounting number of arrests did begin to have an effect on the people who were having to resuscitate most of the victims. Sometime around the last of July or the first of August, in what appears to be one of the first hospital reactions to what was happening several of the ICU nurses approached one of the top medical supervisors—Dr. Duane Freier, pipe-smoking, Harvard-educated chief of surgery—as he made his morning rounds.

The ICU nurses are the most highly trained in the hospital. They are next to doctors in medical knowledge. At night, however, there were usually only a few of them on duty in the unit. As the arrests started mounting they began to find themselves spread thin. They'd no sooner help with one resuscitation than they'd have to run to another. As the arrests increased, they began to worry that there were not enough people to handle them all and that they might have to leave a critically ill patient because of an arrest, and that patient might die.

This was an old complaint. Nurses are always complaining to administration that there aren't enough people to do the job. But in addition to being worried about the overload, the nurses, when they finally decided to talk to Freier, were also beginning to suspect something was wrong. They did not, they say, have even the faintest notion that a poisoner could be at work. But in the back of their minds was another possibility—the arresting patients, most of whom were recently out of surgery, were getting too much, or defective doses of, anesthesia. The majority of the arrests were occurring to patients twenty-four to thirty-six hours post-op, they pointed out.

"By that time," says a male nurse who threatened that he would sue if his name was mentioned, "we had already had eight to twelve arrests close together. That's ridiculous. It doesn't happen in any hospital in that period of time. And the real thing that was bothering us was that they were coming in bunches, and in patients that did not have pulmonary problems and who, before the arrests, seemed to be getting better. You just don't normally see that kind of routine. When you Code 7 three times in one day, four times the next day and two times the day after that, and the numbers keep mounting, you know something is wrong."

But the nurses who approached Freier were day shift nurses, seldom on at night—although sometimes a nursing shortage did require day personnel to stay on at night. They had not worked the bulk of the Code 7s. And so their words appear to have been low-key. In additon, to say that faulty administration of anesthesia might be causing deaths is serious. Without proof, anyone making the accusation is going to be hard pressed to back up what he says. The supposition means error—at least in any normal hospital. Someone will have to be accountable. Reputations and techniques are at stake—possibly careers. There is bound to be resistance to the suggestion.

Freier, a meticulous man, had already, it appears, been alerted to the possibility. No one had yet even conceived that a poisoner could be in operation. The idea, at that time, was practically inconceivable. But another supervisor, Dr. Anne Hill, red-haired, Irish-born head of anesthesiology at the hospital, had begun to become concerned about the arrests too.

As of this writing, Hill has refused to discuss what happened with anyone but official authorities. She did give a couple of press interviews when the fact that a poisoner had been operating in the hospital became public knowledge in mid-August. But that, associates say, was only because her superiors requested her cooperation, thinking it would end press interest in the story. Since then, however, she has steadfastly remained silent. Friends say it is because of professional ethics. In early 1976 she left the country.

But everyone who knows her says Anne Hill is an especially competent and "caring" doctor, more involved with her patients' welfare than the average doctor. Her primary job at the hospital was to oversee the administration of anesthetics and other drugs given to patients in surgery, and then to watch the patients in their recovery periods to see that the process went smoothly.

It was during her watches over some of the recovering patients that she appears to have first been alerted.

One of those patients, her colleagues say, was Emmett J. Lutz, a sixty-two-year-old cancer and emphysema sufferer. Lutz, a farmer from southwest Michigan, had entered the hospital in mid-July. He had a cancerous growth on one of his lungs, and on Friday, July 25, the upper portion of that lung was removed.

Lutz's wife had fretted through the entire operation, an especially long one. But when it was over doctors, she says, assured her it had been a success. The malignancy, they felt, had been removed. She stayed with her husband until he began coming out of the anesthesia. Soon the two were squeezing hands, telling each other, although talking was hard, that everything was all right.

Doctors confirmed that he was recovering well, and by nightfall Mrs. Lutz felt that she could leave. It had been a strenuous day and she was exhausted.

She arrived back at the hospital at 11 A.M. the next day, Saturday, July 26. Almost as soon as she got there, she remembers, there was a respiratory arrest in the ICU—not her husband, but a man in the bed next to him.

Robert Antil, a forty-one-year-old Detroit steelworker and another suspected victim, had an arrest in the ICU on that day at approximately 11:30 A.M. Antil's arrest is probably the one she recalls.

Mrs. Lutz was told that her husband was doing fine, but because of the emergency she'd have to wait a while before seeing him. One of the ICU nurses—the one who threatened to sue if his name was revealed—recalls what happened next:

"I was on the phone talking to a doctor about the earlier arrest. I didn't have any orders on the patient. Mr. Lutz had all the usual post-op stuff around him—tubes, IVs, all that kind of stuff. But everything was looking good for him.

"Suddenly I looked up from the phone and he was seizuring. He was jerking around. His arms were raising and lowering—his eyes rolling. I dropped the phone and shouted, 'What the hell's happening to Mr. Lutz?' Of course, with that, everyone in the unit turned around. And he had stopped breathing.

"He wasn't able to talk by the time I got to him. But he was still shaking. I put an airway in him and started bagging him. I knew it was respiratory because we never lost his heart rate. He always had a cardiac pattern. So it was just a respiratory arrest. By then the code had been called. They intubated him, put him on a respirator, and then everything was fine."

Lutz came right out of the arrest. This was another strange sign. Normally, someone suffering a natural arrest doesn't recover quickly. There usually is a problem that has caused the arrest, and that problem does not go away simply because the patient has been intubated.

But this was at the beginning of the surge of arrests at the end of July, and doctors had not yet had a chance to see, let alone reflect on, the pattern of quick recoveries which would materialize.

Lutz himself doesn't remember a thing about the arrest. In fact, he has a thirteen-day blank in his memory beginning with a few hours before he went into surgery on the twenty-fifth.

The next day, at approximately 6 P.M., doing fine, and apparently for no reason, Lutz, along with another, again arrested.

"They said it could have been the operation," Mrs. Lutz recalls, "but they really didn't know what the reason was."

Since then investigators have positively labeled Lutz's July 27 attack as a murder attempt.

Another of the ICU patients who, Anne Hill's colleagues say, set her to wondering if something might be wrong was Benny Blaine, a forty-six-year-old half Chipewyan construction worker from Ypsilanti, a town next to Ann Arbor.

Blaine was a rotund, crew-cut man who had gone into the hospital July 21 complaining of stomach pains. He had a history of bleeding ulcers and was a heavy drinker, having at least once been treated for alcoholism. The decision was made to rush him immediately into the operating room for exploratory surgery. The operation was a long one. Doctors made an incision in his abdomen from one side to the other. They performed a colostomy—the establishment of an artificial anus by opening a hole in his side and connecting it to the colon. When he finally came out from surgery the diagnosis, according to his large family, which practically lived at the hospital during the time Benny was there, was a blockage in the small intestine.

About a day after surgery Benny's stitches came out—the family says because of incompetence, the hospital says because they were sewed into fat—and he was rushed back into the operating room. Approximately five days later a third thing went wrong—his bowel had been lacerated in the previous operation, his family believes—and again he was rushed back in. By July 29, Blaine was one of the high-priority patients in the ICU, and appropriately in one of the few glass-enclosed single rooms there.

But the last thing in the minds of his doctors was that he would have a respiratory arrest.

Pete Blaine, one of Benny's adult nephews, describes what happened next:

"We were on the fifth floor (two up from the third floor ICU). It was about ten-thirty P.M. A doctor came up and told us Uncle Ben had had an arrest and stopped breathing momentarily. I believe he said for 15 seconds or for a minute and 15 seconds. I can't be sure.

"Somebody asked if that was enough to cause brain damage. The doctor said he didn't think so. Then somebody asked why he'd had the arrest, and the doctor said he didn't know."

Blaine was to experience a second mysterious arrest approximately two weeks later.

By that time, the family was fearful.

Pete recalls:

"It was at night again. This time we were on the third floor by the elevators. You could see the ICU doors. All of a sudden I saw this light on the wall flash with the number 7 on it. I woke my cousin. 'Earl,' I said, 'they've got a respiratory arrest in intensive care.' We knew that's what it was because we'd seen it a lot of times by then. So we started down there.

"There are some windows in the ICU doors and you could see my uncle right across from the nurses' station. He was in a private room. They were pounding on him and sticking things in his throat. And the guy straight across from him, out in the ward, he was having an arrest too. And then a guy to my uncle's left had an arrest. I don't know their names, but they were sticking tubes down them and running around like crazy.

"So we started to go in and they stopped us. They were taking the shock machines down there for the heart. I know about that because I've had rheumatic fever and I've been on these different machines. They were bringing in the big disc machine for shocks. A nurse stopped us and said, 'We've got three emergencies in here and you can't go in.' "

Both times Pete was later allowed in to see his uncle. But Blaine could do no more than look wide-eyed around the room, an intubation tube filling his mouth.

So very probably, Freier, listening to the ICU nurses talking that late July morning when they approached him about the rising number of recent arrests, was already alerted to the strange goings-on. He and Dr. Hill were close. She was his anesthesiologist; he, the chief surgeon. Frequently, after the morning's operations, they would get together over coffee and discuss surgical problems.

And there were others whose cases were puzzling:

Mark H. Hogan, a seventy-five-year-old construction carpenter from Lennon, Michigan, a rural community outside Flint, had been one of those who had arrested on the same night as Benny Blaine, July 29. He would arrest again on August 3.

Hogan was a heart patient. He'd been brought to the hospital on the twenty-ninth. But during his first two arrests, his doctors say, his heart continued to function perfectly. The arrests were clearly respiratory.

In addition, during one or both of the arrests—it is not yet clear, as doctors, too, for several reasons, are reluctant to discuss their patients involved in the case—Hogan's body exhibited an extreme flaccidity, an absence of almost all tone and rigidity. Even dying persons retain a degree of muscle tone until the last moments. But it was as if Hogan's body was completely limp.

Not only is this characteristic of someone who has been given a muscle relaxer, but it is very uncharacteristic of a normal respiratory arrest. When a person stops breathing because of a normal problem, only the diaphragm ceases to work. Hogan apparently lost most, if not all, of his surface muscular function. He must have felt much like the previously mentioned piece of meat in the butcher's hand.

Even more suspicious is the fact that after one of those early arrests, it came to light that Hogan had been fully conscious during one or both of them. The disclosure came in an unexpected way. Although he'd quickly come out of both arrests, which was another indication that they were not normal arrests, he'd had a tube in his mouth and couldn't comment on them. But later, when the tube had been removed and he was being attended by doctors, some of whom had participated in his resuscitation, he recognized a voice.

"I remember you," he is said by a doctor who was present to have suddenly blurted out at one of the surprised physicians. "You're the one who wanted to stop working on me because you thought I was dead."

The allegation was true. One of the doctors had routinely made references to possibly stopping the resuscitation process. But the suggestion had been quickly discarded since there was no evidence of irreparable damage. Hogan's heart monitor, for instance, clearly showed that the heart had not stopped pumping.

This disclosure, however, came some time after the arrest had occurred. Memories had probably clouded. In any case, the other puzzling details of Hogan's problems were not as clear as they had been. No one had put all of the strange aspects together. In addition, Hogan was a very sick man. His arrest could easily be rationalized on that one point alone. Most of the doctors went away feeling that his situation was nothing more than strange—one of those inexplicable things that frequently happen in hospitals.

It is not clear whether Freier was immediately aware of Hogan's case or not. Hogan was not a surgical patient, as were Lutz and Blaine. But Freier was sufficiently concerned about the rising number of arrests to decide to take action.

By late July the hospital's chief of staff, Dr. Martin Lindenauer, had been away from the hospital on sabbatical for several months. In his absence, the various departmental heads had been taking monthly tours as acting chief of staff. Freier's turn was coming up in August. As one of his first official acts he decided to put the problem of the rising arrests on the agenda of the hospital's regular senior staff meeting which was coming up August 4.

Chapter 3

Patients believed to have suffered attacks at the Ann Arbor VA that late July and early August appear, at that time, not to have been aware of precisely what was happening to them. But some were unusually afraid, and did and said things then that when looked back on make their relatives shudder. It is possible, therefore, that a few of the patients might have sensed or known in a confused way that someone might be trying to kill them.

The case of Glenn R. Stout, robust (at least until he got sick) former high school athlete and well-known insurance salesman from Ypsilanti, the town next to Ann Arbor, is illustrative.

Stout, fifty-two, entered the hospital on July 17. He'd had heart problems for the past six months, according to his family, and doctors decided surgery was necessary.

His operation was performed around July 26. When he came out, the family was told everything had gone smoothly except for one thing—a blood clot had formed during the operation and traveled to Stout's big toe, where it had lodged. The toe was turning black, and might have to be removed later.

But the more serious problem had been corrected, they had been assured. Stout had been taken to the ICU and was recovering nicely.

On the twenty-eighth, the day after Emmett Lutz suffered his second unexplainable respiratory arrest, Stout had his first.

The time was approximately 10 P.M. Mrs. Stout recalls: "They had to call me from the hospital. I had gone home thinking he was doing fine. When I got there I never saw anyone with so many tubes. He had three in his arm. He had a bunch of bottles hanging over him. He even had a tube in his mouth. But he came out of the thing real fast. They had some guesses about what had gone wrong, but after tests they said they didn't know why it had happened."

The following day, Stout was well enough to be taken off the respirator. Mrs. Stout had spent the good part of the day with him and by early nightfall felt she could go home without worrying.

"When I got ready to leave," she says, "I said, 'Glenn, I'm going home. Now if you want me, all you have to do is call a nurse and I'll come back.' But he shook his head no and his eyes got real big. And I said, 'Glenn, what's wrong?' All he could do was mumble and I'm not a good lip-reader but I finally figured out that he was saying he was afraid. And I said, 'What are you afraid of?' And he looked at all those tubes, and then his arms. And I said, 'Are you afraid you're going to have another spell like last night?' He nodded yes.

"At that time I didn't think much of it. So much is happening and they're telling you everything is all right. And his hands were tied down so he couldn't make much of a commotion. So I said, 'Well, you're not going to.' And I went over and talked with one of the nurses. I told her he was upset and frightened. And she said, 'We'll take good care of him.'

"But he was petrified," Mrs. Stout says, breaking into sobs and having to stop for a moment. "And when I got home later that night and they called me because he had another spell, I blamed myself. I should have stayed there!"

Again, the arrest came at approximately 10 P.M. This appears to have been the same night Benny Blaine, the heavy half-Chipewyan, and Mark Hogan, the heart patient who remembered hearing his resuscitators, suffered their first attacks, July 29. All three occurred at approximately 10 P.M. Again, the doctors couldn't come up with a good reason for the arrest, says Mrs. Stout. (The hospital today, however, says it wasn't suspicious—but without providing the records to prove it.) And again her husband recovered fast.

By August 2, Stout was doing so well that doctors decided to move him out of the ICU and into the ward at the other end of the third floor.

That night, August 2, was a memorable one at the hospital. Available records indicate there were five arrests, possibly the most that occurred in one day at the hospital in years, and two deaths. Stout was one of the arrests. It was his third mysterious breathing failure in six days. Again, it occurred around 10 P.M. Again, Mrs. Stout, thinking her husband out of danger, had gone home.

"When I got there a man in a wheelchair told me he'd seen it all. Glenn had laid there for a long time [probably asleep] he said, and he [the man observing] hadn't thought anything was wrong. Then all of a sudden everything started to happen. Someone pushed a button and suddenly they were coming out of the woodwork, everybody working on him.

"The doctors said they worked on him for forty-five

minutes. They said they hit him so hard that they broke his ribs. And then they had to open him up and put something in there so he wouldn't puncture his lung. And then they put him back in the ICU and he never came out of it."

Several days later Stout suffered what doctors said was a massive stroke. On August 8, he died.

"The day he died," says Mrs. Stout, "I went in to see him and he was starting to bloat up. They had him on his side. That was the first time they ever moved him as far as I know. I tried to find out what was wrong with him, but nobody answered. Finally, the doctors wouldn't let me back in. They blocked the door. I guess they didn't want me to see him that way. About ten minutes later they came out and told me."

By the time Stout was taken to the morgue, an assorted number of complications and illnesses had been entered onto his chart. Besides his heart problem, he had deteriorating kidneys, and a rupture had been discovered at his brain stem. "Acute lobular pneumonia" was the "primary cause" listed on his death certificate. There wasn't even a mention of the three arrests.

Stout was a sick man, and when the murders and murder attempts would finally be discovered and the doctors would sit down to go over patients' charts to try and discover who had been victims and who had not, he would not be placed high on the list. His fears probably wouldn't even have been considered and it is doubtful the doctors would even have known about them, being, by then, far removed from the actual incident. It is not uncommon for ICU patients to express fear, or even paranoia.

But Stout's family, until shown proof to the contrary, will probably always believe he was a victim. The three unexplained arrests—all at approximately the same time—are just too coincidental for them to believe otherwise. And Mrs. Stout, whose recollections of those late July and early August days are corroborated in substance by her two adult sons, will probably always blame herself for not staying in the hospital the night of her husband's second arrest—not that it would have done any good.

Evidence indicates that the presence of persons near the victims did not deter the killer.

Another believed victim who might have been aware of something was Harold VanDenBerg, a retired railroad man living on his sister's farm near Battle Creek.

VanDenBerg, sixty-nine, a tall, lanky man, had a pacemaker, a small electrical machine that stimulates heart contractions, in his chest. On August 2 something went wrong with the pacemaker and he collapsed while working outside. He was sufficiently recovered in time, however, says his family, to be able to direct the out-of-town ambulance to the VA once it reached Ann Arbor.

Admitted to the VA, VanDenBerg was immediately put in the ICU and hooked up to support machines. By that night, says his son, an Army sergeant, the decision to move him out of intensive care and into a ward for less seriously ill patients had already been made. He was in the ICU only for observation.

At approximately 11:30 P.M., however, VanDenBerg suffered an unexpected breathing failure. "The doctors said for 'no apparent reason.' That's a direct quote," says his son. August 2 was the night of five arrests. VanDenBerg was probably the fifth, shortly after Stout.

"I got there the next day," says the son, who runs a radar maintenance crew in northern Michigan. "They didn't seem to know any particulars about how it happened. They seemed stumped. But they were definite in calling it a respiratory arrest. His heart was doing fine.

"I couldn't talk to Dad because he had a tube in his mouth. But he seemed apprehensive. He'd look around. You know, like when you're afraid of something, kind of wide-eyed like. I got the impression—and my wife got the impression—that he was trying to say something to us. But, of course, he couldn't talk. He'd get excited and his machine would go crazy. It sounded as if he was coughing into it.

"At the time I thought it was a combination of the shock of what had happened to him and then being in a strange place. But now I don't know. Dad's mind is a blank about all this. He's got a two-week gap. But when he finally woke up, he was very indignant about his hands being all taped up. They had taped cotton over his hands, they said, because he'd tried to pull the IVs out of his arms.

"Now my dad's been in the hospital a lot of times. He's had several serious operations and lots of IVs in him. And he's never before tried to pull IVs out of his arms. The thing that leaps to my mind is, did he suspect?"

Unlike Stout, VanDenBerg would be placed high on all the suspicious lists when the hospital finally found out what was going on and called the FBI.

But no lists had been drawn up by August 4—the date on which, it appears, the hospital for the first time considered the mounting number of arrests in a senior staff meeting, a meeting of many of the hospital's leaders. Hospital officials had not even determined that the arrests were suspicious. They seemed, as already shown, simply puzzling. However, Dr. Freier, by then acting chief of staff—the one who, after consultations with Anne Hill, had decided to place the rising arrest rate on the meeting's agenda—had become more concerned about the arrests than he had been earlier.

The five arrests on August 2 must have made an impression. In addition, when Freier took over as chief on August 1, he suddenly was presented with a much larger picture.

"In late July, we were dealing only with surgical patients and with isolated cases," he says. "Taken alone, they didn't make such an impact. The hospital was full and we had an awful lot of people who were extremely ill. But beginning August 1, I started a morning report [presumably where the previous night's arrests were listed]. I began seeing what was happening in the rest of the hospital. I found out that the medicine people [those on the other large service in the hospital] were having the same problems we [surgery] were. Then it became obvious that things were getting unusual."

The medicine service was headed by Dr. Ronald Bishop, bow tie-wearing, long time staffer at the VA, and a local civic leader. In 1969, Bishop had been elected to the Ann Arbor school board. He was active at Ann Arbor's First Unitarian Church, and was a former member of the American Civil Liberties Union's local executive board.

Bishop, too, was unaware at this time that anything sinister was going on. In late July he had been approached by the respiratory therapists whose job it was to maintain and operate the mechanical respirators in the hospital and aid in intubations. The therapists are under the medicine service. They, like the nurses who had approached Freier, had complained of understaffing. The rising number of arrests was irritating an already bad situation, they had told Bishop. They wanted more people.

But Bishop had not fully understood what was going on. "I associated their appeal to me with the normal complaints," he says. "Understaffing was a chronic complaint. We always needed more therapists. The fact is we didn't have enough money. But I felt it was my duty to pass on the complaint. So I took it to the administration. I can't remember exactly who. But I have to admit I considered it somewhat routine. I knew we'd had more arrest activity, but I didn't realize there was anything more to it."

So Bishop had been aware of the rising number of arrests, but he had not had direct daily patient contact which might have caused him to become alarmed. Most of the arrests, as already pointed out, were occurring to surgery, not medicine, patients.

The minutes of the August 4 meeting are locked away somewhere in the hospital. The administrator's office to date won't even volunteer how many suspicious arrests occurred, let alone allow outside access to official records. But it is not hard, with the aid of interviews with some of the participants, to paint a picture of what probably went on. The gist has already been made public.

August 4 was a Monday. Those there remember it was hot at that time. The doctors, probably still somewhat relaxed from the weekend (Freier is an avid tennis player and jogger, and Bishop rides his bicycle "when the weather is good"), filed into an air-conditioned boardroom and took chairs at a large table. It was probably just after lunch (most of the meetings were held at that time), and idle talk was exchanged until everyone was settled.

The meeting's official title was "Clinical Executive Board Meeting." It was a regular occurrence at the hospital every two weeks. Lower staffers met weekly in their respective departments. In addition to Freier and Bishop, Anne Hill, supervisory doctors from other services and members of the non-medical administration were present. Freier presided. The meetings usually lasted from an hour to an hour and a half.

After some preliminary business, the arrests were

most likely discussed, with Drs. Freier and Hill voicing their suspicions. Dr. Hill may have gone into specific cases and the fact that at this point the only common denominators as yet solidly established were that almost all the arrests were occurring at night, and all the victims appeared to have been on intravenous solutions. The possibility of contamination accidents from defective equipment, wrong—or even bad—medicine could have been raised

It may have been at this point that Bishop would have spoken. He recalls saying something resembling the following: "I don't know about any contamination, but I do know that we need more respiratory therapists. Just this week they came to me and said as much. The rising arrests are putting a terrible strain on them. They need help—maybe as many as five more therapists. Right now we only have three on at night.

"I know we've only got so much money, but I wonder if priorities were perhaps shifted to the respiratory unit, might not this arrest rate go down? After all, they're in the thick of it. If they had more help, maybe we wouldn't have so many arrests."

Months later, Bishop did say, "I think as you look back what I said was a little irrational. I was actually using the situation to emphasize our needs. And it was not an appropriate response. But none of us at that time really knew what was going on."

Bishop's remarks were probably considered and then the main issue returned to. An account prepared for a University of Michigan journal says a member of the non-medical administration gave some statistics: the fact that the hospital's normal rate of arrests was six to eight per month, and that currently that rate was about six times as high. Dr. Freier's approach appears to have been cautious. The Detroit *Free Press*, later reporting about the meeting, quotes him as saying, "I just put it to them. I said, 'I'm new at this and I need some advice. Should we go ahead with a formal investigation of all this?' "

A formal investigation would mean public knowledge of a potentially embarrassing situation and the probable stepping in of outside authorities. There appears to have been resistance to the investigation suggestion. "This can be a terrible headache and I don't believe we need the bad publicity," somebody might have said. "Besides," he might have added correctly, "nothing is concrete. We really don't know what we have. Contamination is a serious and improbable thing. It might simply be coincidence. We have an unusually high number of sick patients in the hospital, and everybody knows these kinds of problems multiply in the summer. I think, for now, we should handle this ourselves."

Bishop says, "There is no question that we were concerned about the arrests. But the thing we were concerned about was, were *we* doing something wrong? Was there some medication being administered that shouldn't be used? It was a self-examination as much as anything else."

The discussion, according to all reports, lasted only a short time. The group then went on to other business. The suggestion of a formal investigation was shelved. Instead, Anne Hill was asked to begin a systematic review of the medical charts of all the patients involved. Hopefully, she would uncover something previously overlooked. Perhaps in an hour the meeting was adjourned. Murder, according to all available evidence, was still inconceivable—something for books or movies, but certainly not a professional hospital. Contamination was the most serious consideration, and it was only a remote possibility.

Still no one suspected.

Chapter 4

The Ann Arbor VA nurses, a relatively close-knit group, undoubtedly were the hardest hit of all the hospital's medical personnel by the mounting arrests. At night there were only a few of them on duty, usually two registered nurses in the ICU (along with assistants), and perhaps one RN (along with possibly one assistant) per floor. Even when things were going smoothly, these night staffers had their hands full. They had to give out medications, change dressings at regular intervals, make periodic bed and room checks and complete always accumulating paper work. Even one unexpected arrest would throw their tight schedule completely out of whack.

"We were already short-staffed," recalls one, "and when the doctors got through they'd leave you with a patient that hopefully is alive, but probably a total mess. Maybe they've started an IV on them. So you've got blood all over the sheets. Maybe the patient urinated during the arrest, so you've got a wet bed. You've got all kinds of broken vials around. It's just a catastrophe in that room. And you've got to clean it up. The doctors make a note on the patient's chart, walk off, and that's the end of it for them. Your work is just beginning."

And whereas a doctor's training and knowledge usually gave him a measure of control during a crisis, a nurse was less likely to be calm. Sometimes, in peak stress situations, the frantic work and feeling of helplessness caused anxiety, even near panic. On at least one night of heavy activity, two nurses are known to have become ill—one actually fainting—in the midst of a fast-breaking string of arrests.

"I remember one night," recalls another nurse, "we'd no sooner started working on a patient at one end of a wing than another arrest was called at the other end. We had to drop the first and run to the second. And it went on and on like that." Still another nurse told the Detroit *Free Press*, "I can't describe how terrible it was. Night afer night after night you'd see that 7 flashing."

The nurses are hard to question. They are suspicious of almost everyone. But those who have gained their confidence say eating during late July and early August became almost a luxury. There was seldom ever enough time. Exhaustion and irritability became commonplace. The nurses knew something was wrong, but, to them, their complaints seemed to fall on deaf ears. They were not it appears, privy to the high-level conferences at which the problem had begun to be discussed.

Eventually things became so bad that some nurses, it is said, even threatened to quit. There's no question that many of them began to dread coming in at night. One of these nurses was Denise Nichol, a petite, brown-haired former "Trojet" one of a group of dancing baton twirlers that performed between halves at her high school athletic events and a graduate of the University of Michigan nursing school.

According to her mother, Denise, twenty-two, was an outgoing, energetic girl who loved swimming and had many friends. Photos show her with large brown eyes behind thick, black eyelashes. She had wanted to be a nurse from the time she was a little girl, and so her job at the VA was a happy one—until late July 1975.

At that time, say her friends, she became caught up in the mounting arrests. "She would call or see me at least once a day," recalls her mother. "She said they were having an extraordinary amount of codes and she talked about having to go to so many."

Denise worked on the sixth floor, but because of the understaffing, says her mother, she was often called to other floors to help out. As a result, Denise was concerned that the patients she had to leave were unattended, and wrote her superior that she would quit if something wasn't done about the situation. The superior, a doctor, was finally reached in Utah, where he had moved by early 1976. But he hung up the phone with a terse "I'm no longer connected to that situation," when reached long-distance. So the existence of the letter could not be confirmed.

By early August, say her friends, it was noticed that Denise and many of the arrests were somehow associated. Some say that wherever Denise went, a patient seemed to stop breathing. Others say simply that she was present at many of the resuscitations. To relieve tension, some of the nurses joked about this. But Denise, a sensitive girl, according to all accounts, became upset. One day, it is reported, she turned to a friend and said, "Maybe I should get out of nursing. I feel like a jinx." Her friends, however, assured her everything was all right.

But then a mysterious thing happened. On August 7, in the middle of the mounting arrests, Denise, who had been as close to them as anyone, was found dead in her apartment, directly across the street from the hospital. She was propped up on her bed, legs hanging over the side, facing a television with the picture and sound on. A bottle of Darvon, a pain-killer, was on the night table beside her. A lighted cigarette and glass of wine had fallen from her fingers. The cigarette had smoldered for a while, burning a small hole in the rug. The wine was spilled. It was as if she'd suddenly slumped dead. There was no sign of struggle; no suicide note. The alarm on her bedside clock was pulled out, as if she had intended to get up in the morning.

On August 7, however, what was going on at the hospital had not yet been discovered. Police were not aware that there might be any connection. They investigated the death routinely. At first the cause was officially listed as "undetermined pending investigation." There were certain puzzling aspects. It was assumed Denise had died of an overdose of the Darvon. She was menstruating, and had complained of cramps. But the amount of the pain-killer in her bloodstream was not considered a lethal dose. Then, two months later, after the hospital murders had come to light, and there had been speculation that Denise's death had somehow been linked, the official cause of death was changed to "accidental."

Darvon is a much stronger drug than is commonly known, the investigators are said to have found out. Denise was also a small girl. A little bit might have been more lethal to her. It probably was an overdose, they concluded. It certainly wasn't suicide. The death was just a tragic accident—a strange coincidence with the hospital murders—but nothing more.

However, a small group of Denise's nursing friends, who by then were aware of the hospital attacks, were convinced that she had been murdered. The reason, they believed, was that Denise might have known something about the killer or killers. Being present at so many arrests, she might have seen something. One of the nurses is said to have told reporters that just a few days before her death Denise had tried to tell her something that seemed urgent. The two were in one of the hospital's halls, the nurse is said to have recalled, but Denise was stopped short by the sudden appearance of a third person the nurses now think may have been involved in the hospital deaths.

And there were unanswered questions about Denise's death that fed their conviction:

Shortly after Denise had moved into her apartment, she had been entertaining relatives at dinner when someone had unexpectedly opened the front door from the hall and walked in. Denise had thought the door was locked. The incident scared her, and she had bought a latch lock that could only be fastened from the inside.

Ever since that incident, friends and relatives said she had religiously locked the latch each time she had entered the apartment or let someone else out.

It was a conspicuous quirk.

But the day she was found dead, the latch was not locked. The conclusion her friends came to was that somebody other than Denise had been the last through the door, and that Denise had not been able to fasten the latch herself. She had been dead or dying by that time.

Also, if Denise had died of Darvon overdose, why wasn't there a sign of at least a little disturbance in the room? Presumably, a lethal overdose is preceded by movement of some sort while the victim becomes progressively sicker. Wouldn't she have vomited, tried to put her cigarette down or at least have made an attempt to get up? On the other hand, the seeming lack of a struggle—the fact, for instance, that the television was still on when she was found, which led investigators to believe that she had been unsuspectingly watching it when whatever killed her struck suddenly—fit a Pavulon death exactly.

She might have moved her arms or legs a bit, but the available evidence indicates she dropped almost in her tracks.

Had someone injected Denise with a muscle relaxer and then left through the front door undetected?

Such questions arose mostly from speculation. But the fact that both the crime scene search and Denise's autopsy were performed before anyone knew about the Pavulon deaths at the VA justified the asking of them. Had anybody checked Denise's body for needle marks? Had the wine she was drinking, and the wineglass, been analyzed?

These questions were primary in the minds of persons who, after the VA deaths had been discovered, went back over Denise's death and were struck by some of its peculiarities. But the authorities—the Ann Arbor police who did the initial investigation into her death, and the pathologist who performed the autopsy—refused to answer them. The case is private and closed, was their response to all outside inquiries. And they ridiculed the inquirers for questioning their findings.

One of the persons, however, who listened intently to the speculation was Denise's mother. In fact, she, for a time, questioned the official findings as well.

The Nichol home, in an affluent development twenty miles outside Ann Arbor, was large and ranch-type. It sat on the top of a hill. Denise had a large family. Her mother and father were crushed by the death. Months later they were still running the details through their minds, hoping to figure it out, not understanding why it happened. Denise was very close to both of them.

"She would call or see me at least once a day," recalls her mother. "About a week or so before she died she said they were having an extraordinary amount of codes, and she talked about having to go to so many ... I don't think it's impossible that she could have been murdered because of something she knew. Some of her friends think so. They've been to see us several times."

Denise was upset on the night she died, says Mrs. Nichol—but not, as far as her mother knew, because of anything concerning the arrests.

"On that afternoon a lawyer had come to talk to her at the hospital. [She had worked the day shift August 6.] An Ann Arbor inn had burned down, I believe, and the man [accused of doing it] had been a patient of hers. The lawyer wanted her to testify about the patient's sanity. She'd never had anything to do with courts and I guess she was afraid. She wasn't a doctor and she didn't want to testify about the patient's mental state."

Because she was upset, says her mother, a couple of the nurses she worked with took her for a drink at the lounge in her apartment building, a place frequented by employees of the hospital as well as by young singles from all over Ann Arbor. They had a few drinks, but when the other girls suggested going to more lounges, Denise declined.

The period cramps were bothering her and she felt like going up to her apartment, says her mother. At about 6:30 P.M. she called home.

"She told me all about the lawyer, and I said don't worry. She remarked she'd have to be in court on her birthday, August 20. She wasn't real upset. Denise was the type who could get upset real easily but then calm down quickly. She was just complaining about it and I soothed her."

The only thing Mrs. Nichol knows about what happened in the next five or six hours is that Denise had a visitor. The identity of the visitor cannot be revealed because of possible future developments in Denise's death.

Mrs. Nichol says she knows Denise admitted the visitor because at approximately 12:15 A.M. Denise called her back and told her. She (Denise) was not as upset as before about the lawyer. But she had a new problem: a disagreement she and the visitor had had. Although the visitor has a connection to the VA, the problem, as far as Mrs. Nichol knows, had nothing to do with the VA arrests. It was social.

The visitor had left at around midnight, says Mrs. Nichol, but at the time, she says, she did not attach much significance to the visit or the time.

"When she signed off, another thing she talked about was the cramps. She didn't feel good. And when she was ready to hang up she said she wasn't sleepy and she felt like she was going to watch TV for a while. I said you better not stay up too late because you've got to go to work in the morning. So she said she wouldn't. She said she'd watch for a little while just to get sleepy. She said bye, 'I'll talk to you tomorrow.' And that was it."

At approximately 1:30 A.M., says Mrs. Nichol, Denise called into the VA saying she had a "severe headache" and didn't think she'd be coming into work the next morning, "but if she felt better she would."

It must be hard, today, for Mrs. Nichol to reconcile in her mind that at approximately 1:30 A.M. Denise appeared unaware of any Darvon coma coming on and then by 2 A.M. she is believed to have been dead from it.

Police theorize, says Mrs. Nichol, that the time of death was probably before 2 A.M. This is because, she says, since the station Denise was watching went off at 2 A.M., had Denise been awake and well at the time she probably would have turned it off or at least changed stations.

"She was sitting on the bed as if watching the TV when I found her," Mrs. Nichol says.

No one, as far as available evidence indicates, ever spoke to Denise after 1:30 A.M., August 7.

At approximately 9:30 A.M. the next morning, says Mrs. Nichol, she received a phone call from the visitor who had been at Denise's the night before. The visitor said several attempts to reach Denise by phone that morning had failed.

Prompted by the call, Mrs. Nichol says she then began phoning Denise herself. No answer. At around noon, she says, she started getting worried. It was then she called the hospital and found out that Denise had called in sick at 1:30 A.M. About 3 P.M., August 7, Mrs. Nichol says she was "really upset," and decided to go over to the apartment herself to see if anything was wrong.

"I drove over and knocked on the door. No answer. I called. No answer. So I went down to the office and got the girl there and told her I didn't have a key and would she please let me in.

"As she was getting ready to unlock the door she said, 'Oh, if the inside lock is on we won't be able to go in.' At the time, I didn't think much of it, but the lock *wasn't* on. It was unlocked. Denise always kept the lock on.

"So I unlocked the door and the girl waited at the door for me. She didn't go in. And I walked in and went back toward the bedroom. And I could see that the TV was still on. When I went into the bedroom I found her. And I touched her to see ... I felt like when I saw her that way that she was dead, but I'd never found anyone dead so I touched her to be sure.

"I guess I just started screaming and the girl from the office came in."

The police checked several of the puzzles surrounding Denise's death but, after the two-month interval of investigation, finally decided that the evidence was mostly in favor of an accidental overdose. A sad coincidence for the family was that Denise's father was a pharmaceutical salesman. Mindful of his daughter's nurse training, which included instruction on how to use drugs, he must have wondered why she, of all people, could have died that particular way.

"But she was not careful with her health," he says. "She hadn't eaten all day, maybe not for thirty-six hours. And so you know then that the Darvon would have gone right into her bloodstream. Maybe she took two for the cramps, then two more, and then two more later—without even thinking about it. According to the pathologist, her dropping of the cigarette could be explained by her becoming drowsy and it falling out of her hand."

After the murders and murder attempts had been discovered at the VA, and Denise's part in the resuscitations learned, the FBI—which, since the hospital is in a federal enclave, has jurisdiction in the Pavulon deaths—contacted the Ann Arbor police to review the case. But their main interest was in finding the VA killer or killers, according to a federal lawman involved in the investigation. And because the murder attempts continued after Denise's death, they decided not to pursue the nurse's case any further.

If she was not the killer, then they already had enough mystery on their hands, was probably their thinking.

In time, after continually questioning the police and the pathologist, and continually being told that they were only torturing themselves worrying about puzzles that only the press and a few others felt consequential, the Nichol family, too, decided to accept the official findings.

"It's a possibility that Denise was murdered," conceded her father in January 1976. "But then it does seem coincidental that she also would have a lethal dose of Darvon in her bloodstream."

Although reporters, without the official reports, had never been able to accept that, Mr. Nichol finally did.

"The nurses came to see us again this Sunday, and we started the questioning again. But my wife then talked to the pathologist Monday and he assured her it was a lethal dose.

"We've been crushed. It's been a different world since Denise left. I never thought I'd experience anything like it. Our whole life had been built around our children. Maybe now we'll get around to the point where we won't cry ourselves to sleep every night."

Chapter 5

Following the flurry of suspicious arrests at the end of July and the first few days of August, a strange, ominous calm appears to have descended over the Ann Arbor VA. Available figures are unofficial, perhaps faulty, but it's possible there was only one code called between the fourth and the eighth of August. There definitely were fewer than in the previous week.

Had the killer or killers taken a holiday? Had he or she or they decided to lay low after so many earlier attacks?

No one, at least publicly as of this writing, has given any answers (if there are any) to such questions. But one thing seems certain: no one outside the hospital at that time suspected anything at all out of the ordinary was occurring inside it. Two days following the discovery of Denise Nichol's body, for instance, the Ann Arbor *News*, the local area's largest newspaper, listed Denise and Glenn Stout (the Ypsilanti insurance man whose wife believes he might have known he was in danger) in its regular "Deaths" column without the slightest indication the two might have been linked.

In fact, the newspaper, a check of its back issues

shows, appears to have run nothing but stories praising the VA hospital for years previous.

At the VA itself, however, the atmosphere ranged from stark fear in some of the nurses to rising apprehension in a few of the senior doctors. (Most of the younger doctors still suspected nothing.) "It was one of those deep-seated uneasy feelings that you don't have things under control," Dr. Freier later told a reporter.

The day before Denise Nichol's death, the surgical staff had conducted one of its Death and Complications conferences, a weekly meeting where matters of concern to the surgeons were discussed. The mounting arrests had already come up at one previous conference, and a particular arrest victim became the focus of this meeting.

Dr. Freier, who presided, says there are no minutes of the meeting because they were usually informal affairs. But he agrees that it's very possible that Mark Hogan, who had exhibited a strange flaccidity during his arrests and, surprisingly, had heard his resuscitators working over him, could have been the patient. "His certainly was one of the most puzzling cases," Freier volunteers.

But as the surgeons isolated the case, its strangeness, Freier adds, seemed to vanish.

Hogan was in extremely poor health. Even if he hadn't been, at seventy-five, he was a prime candidate for complications. He had a history of cardiac arrest, and every doctor knows it's common for breathing stoppages to follow heart attacks. Even the peculiarity of his seemingly feeling good, having a sudden arrest and then snapping right out of it was not so unusual, the doctors could have concluded. He'd done it several times before, the records that were probably before them would have indicated.

In addition, Hogan, according to his wife (and it can be assumed the doctors would have been aware of the fact also), had emphysema. Emphysema is a lung disease. Doctors faced with an unexplainable respiratory problem would logically view the emphysema as a possible cause.

And so if it had been Hogan whom the surgeons had dwelled upon August 6, it is understandable that his poor health could have obscured the puzzling aspects of his arrest (or arrests)—especially in light of the probable fact that the number of arrests at the hospital seemed to be dropping.

Rather than being pressed by mounting codes, the doctors were probably beginning to feel a little relieved at the sudden decline, and maybe even that they'd perhaps been a little hasty in suspecting the worst—a contamination accident.

But it wasn't long before they were jolted back to reality.

Most probably on August 8 (the date is not positively certain yet), there was another rash of arrests. Not a great rash. The number appears to have been three, all in the ICU. Hogan, again, may have been among them. All appear to have occurred during what is officially referred to as the afternoon shift—that is, the shift that runs from 4 P.M. to midnight, and can also be called the evening shift.

One of the patients who appears to have been attacked that night is William Loesch, a Detroit-area Vietnam veteran in his mid-twenties who would become important in the investigation of the case.

According to his mother, Loesch had served in the Marine Corps during some of the heavy fighting in Vietnam. But she couldn't remember the particulars. "He was in the front lines with tanks and big guns," she says. "I would probably have the name of his unit in some of his letters, but right offhand, I can't remember it." Loesch himself could not be contacted. He had moved from his Ann Arbor address by late 1975, and even his mother didn't know where he was. (Although she may have just been reluctant to disclose his whereabouts. He is said to fear for his safety because of what happened to him in the VA.)

Loesch, according to doctors and nurses who attended him, was admitted to the VA sometime in July with a gunshot wound. The bullet had penetrated his liver. He was in the ICU recovering from surgery when he suffered the August 8 arrest. Since he couldn't be reached, and his mother, after talking a short while, decided she didn't want to continue, not much is known about the arrest. But several weeks after hospital officials discovered the Pavulon killings and Loesch was subsequently identified as one of the surviving victims, a Detroit *Free Press* reporter, Jim Schutze, obtained an exclusive interview with him by agreeing to conceal in his article Loesch's identity.

The following is largely from that interview, which was published in the *Free Press* September 4, 1975, and subsequently carried by other papers across the country.

Being injected with Pavulon "feels like instant death," Loesch told Schutze. "It's just like somebody grabbed hold of your throat real quick. And it's just how long you can hold your breath—maybe thirty, maybe sixty seconds. Then your whole body goes numb.

"It hits the vision first," Loesch, who eventually suffered three arrests, continued. "Your right eye goes way to the right. Your left eye goes way to the left. Then you feel nausea. The first time . . . everything just slowly stopped. But the last time was really bad."

Loesch was asleep when the August 8 attack occurred, he told Schutze. He had an IV in his arm. The IV needle was attached to a tube leading to a clear plastic bag. Usually, near the top of the tube there's a rubber coupling device—a small brown apparatus which nurses and doctors use to introduce medications. The rubber won't sprout a leak when a needle is stuck into it as the plastic tubing might.

It was into this small brown coupling device that investigators believe Loesch's attacker injected the Pavulon.

Describing a later arrest, Loesch told Schutze: "I felt a pain in my IV." He rolled over and the effects were on him in a matter of seconds. "My whole body felt like it went up in flames, and that was it." The next thing he remembered, according to the article, was waking up surrounded by doctors and nurses who told him that he was lucky to be alive.

It is not known whether Loesch told any of this to the doctors who attended his August 8 arrest. Most probably he did not. He likely thought the strange and unnerving experience the result of his condition. It probably wasn't until the murders were discovered nearly a week later that he realized what had happened.

But even if he had, the doctors probably would have discounted his claims as the fantasy of a paranoid ICU patient. Loesch had some personal problems, he told Schutze, and claims of tortuous medicines were not infrequent in the eerie ICU.

But Loesch's arrest—the August 8 arrest, at least—was nothing compared to what was to come. For the shaky calm at the hospital was soon to explode into an eruption of arrests and deaths unlike any at the hospital before.

Four nights after Loesch's August 8 arrest, there

were to be an incredible eight codes called at the hospital in a span of less than four hours.

The early August calm, it appears, was a lull before a storm.

Chapter 6

The ICU had a scrubbed and polished look. Dr. Thomas Weber, a fifth-year surgery resident, was working overtime, attending to some patients. It was late in the afternoon. Tuesday, August 12. The number of arrests had begun to pick up again. On August 10, there appears to have been at least one; on August 11, at least two. Weber was aware of the arrest problem. As a senior surgery resident he had been one of those talking with Dr. Hill and Dr. Freier. They had informed him of the contamination possibility, and he had been participating in the chart review initiated at the senior staff meeting August 4.

But the problem was still not of paramount concern to him. Two of his patients, Benny Blaine and Emmett Lutz, had suffered several of the most puzzling arrests. But he really did not yet believe that there was anything more involved than the unexplained events that sometimes occur in acute care situations.

He was not expecting what was about to happen.

Dr. Dennis Penner, upstairs on the seventh floor checking pulmonary patients, was even less expectant.

A first-year resident in internal medicine, Penner's

schedule was such that only once before had he served as the MOD (medical officer of the day—one of only two physicians officially on duty that night). He had participated in one resuscitation, but that had been several weeks before. Not being a surgeon, even the discussions of the puzzling patients were far removed from him.

As he recalls it, he too had no idea of anything approximating what was going to happen.

And Penner wasn't looking forward to his all-night duty either. He had just finished a full day on his regular 8 A.M. to 4 P.M. shift. Following the MOD duty, he would be required to serve a third shift without a break. At most other hospitals according to Penner, a doctor working two shifts back to back would usually get relief. But not at the VA, and he accepted it without complaint.

In addition, Penner, twenty-seven, from Detroit, was AOD that night—administrative officer of the day. This meant that along with his medical duties, he had to attend to all the administrative problems that came up.

Even if the night had remained uneventful, Penner would have had his hands full.

The first arrest occurred in the ICU at approximately 5:45 P.M.

"As I remember," says Dr. Weber, "I was checking over one of my patients when a nurse yelled cardiac arrest or Code 7. It wasn't the patient I was attending, so I ran over." The victim was Benny Blaine, who had suffered a suspicious arrest in late July. He was in one of the unit's private, glass-enclosed rooms. When he got to him, says Weber, Blaine was "unresponsive."

"One of the first things you do when a code is called is deliver several blows on the chest. But as I remember the patient was hooked up to a cardiac monitor and we could see that he had a heartbeat of some sort. So while someone else started closed-chest massage, because we still didn't know what his blood pressure was, I immediately put a tube in him and started bagging. As I remember we soon found that he had good blood pressure. We knew he had a good pulse. His problem was that he couldn't breathe."

Upstairs, Penner heard the code broadcast over his pocket beeper. He dropped what he was doing and took off for the stairs leading to the ICU. But he had four floors to dash down, and by the time he got there, Blaine was already starting to stabilize.

"I asked them if there was anything I could do," he recalls. "but they said they had everything under control."

Blaine was recovering from a serious operation on August 12, but his problems were abdominal, not pulmonary. As after his first arrest, July 29, there didn't seem to be any medical reason why he had suddenly stopped breathing.

But the doctors didn't have much time to consider that fact, for as they watched Blaine recovering, a second code was called.

The second arrest was out in the ICU's open ward, a group of beds arranged around the wall at the end of the unit. Again, a nurse called it. The particular patient was in a bed approximately thirty feet from where the doctors stood. His name was Larry Richards, a forty-three-year-old project engineer for Cadillac who, like Blaine, had undergone stomach surgery.

To see Richards, all the doctors had to do was turn around. The glass windows surrounding Blaine's room gave them a view of that area of the ward. And what they saw was highly unusual.

Richards was approximately half up in his bed "gesturing to his throat," recalls Penner. "He couldn't talk, but his arms were moving. It was like he was trying to tell us he couldn't breathe. Mostly I remember his arms."

The doctors immediately ran over.

"He had this anxious look on his face," says Weber, "and I yelled to him, 'Take a breath!' But he just kept pointing to his throat."

Suddenly Richards went limp. Weber thought maybe he had an obstruction in his throat. "He had a nasogastric tube in place and I thought maybe it had gotten coiled up." But thrusting his fingers down Richards' gullet, the surgeon felt nothing.

By then the "crash cart" had been wheeled to the bedside, and Richards was intubated. "His pulse and blood pressure were fine through the whole thing," says Weber. "It was just a matter of getting him ventilated and he was all right."

Afterward, when Richards was sufficiently revived to talk (maybe even several days later), Weber asked him what had happened. "He said, 'I don't know. All of a sudden I just couldn't breathe.'" He didn't know anything else.

Richards' arrest was as puzzling as was Blaine's right before him. But at the time it appeared to be just a coincidence.

At approximately 6:30 P.M., with Richards stabilized and, as Penner recalls, "the group of us talking about what the hell was that," the third code was called.

The victim this time was William Loesch, the young Vietnam veteran with the gunshot wound who had arrested for the first time on August 8, four days earlier. Loesch was in the ICU's other glass-enclosed room. It was right next to Blaine's, only closer to the ICU entrance. Both private rooms were off the ICU hallway leading from the entrance to the open ward. Both were right across from the nurse's station.

Again, a nurse was the first to spot the arrest say the doctors. They immediately ran back.

"He was just kind of lying there staring straight up at the ceiling with his eyes wide open and not breathing," recalls Weber. "He was out and he was blue," says Penner. The two, with the help of others there, intubated him. Again, the victim quickly recovered.

In roughly forty-five minutes, there had now been three breathing arrests, almost one right after the other. Weber, the older and more experienced of the two, was beginning to get suspicious—not of foul play, he says, but of a contamination accident. "The suspicions I'd heard were suddenly in my mind, and I guess I began to think there must be something in the IV bottles. What had happened just didn't make sense."

Penner, however, thought at least he might have an explanation for Loesch's arrest: "He had arrested before, and I remembered the last time, he had had fluid in his chest from the gunshot wound and other problems. I didn't remember the details of his case. I just knew he had a lot of fluid and people thought maybe that was the reason. So I figured, well, maybe the same thing happened again."

But Penner, too, was beginning to sense irregularity, and not just because of the three arrests close together. Arrests usually are caused by serious internal problems. Patients suffering them are hard to revive. Normal hospital resuscitation rates are around 30 per cent successful, or less. And when the patient is revived he often is unstable. But he and Weber were experiencing a 100 per cent resuscitation rate. They were three for three, and none of the patients had any post-arrest problems.

But the younger doctor didn't have much time to

contemplate this, for by the time Loesch was stabilized, a problem arose on the first floor in admitting, and as AOD, Penner had to attend to it. Weber, still mulling over what had happened, and consequently preferring silence about his suspicions, stayed on in the ICU.

There was a lull of about forty-five minutes, and then at approximately 7:45 P.M. a fourth code was called.

The patient was in the open ward again, several beds away from Richards, the second arrest that night. An old man, the fourth arrest victim had serious lung disease and had just been moved to the ICU because of a rapidly worsening condition.

Weber recalls: "As I remember I wasn't that surprised about him. He had bad emphysema. He had bad blood gases [a result of the emphysema]. But he was wide awake when it happened. He was a little mentally questionable at the time and had been babbling to himself. All of a sudden somebody noticed he wasn't talking anymore. When they went over to check him, he wasn't breathing."

Penner, also not surprised at the old man's arrest, heard the code over his pocket beeper and dashed back up. "When they got to him he had the full arrest—no heart rhythm, no respiration. I don't know the sequence—which came first—but he required bagging and an injection of bicarbonate and epinephrine [adrenaline] to get his heart rhythm back."

After resuscitation, the old man was still unstable. Penner, who then took over, had to do more work on him. One of the first things was to give him a larger IV so medicines needed would travel faster. The new IV was to go underneath the clavicle in the upper chest. Penner had just inserted the needle when unbelievably a fifth code was sounded.

This arrest, however, was unlike the others. The patient next to the old man was already hooked up to a mechanical respirator. Aware of the activity beside him, he'd become excited and yanked his tube out. Although it wasn't that serious, one of the doctors still had to detach himself from the resuscitation in progress and put the tube back.

The fourth and fifth resuscitations took about half an hour. By the time they were done, it was approximately 8:15 P.M. way past dinner time, and Penner and Weber were exhausted. They had gone from resuscitation to resuscitation practically non-stop. Five arrests in one day, let alone in two hours, was almost unheard of. They were drained emotionally and physically. Weber, however, was lucky. Not on official duty, he could go home. Penner, MOD and AOD had to stay.

At home, given a respite and time to think, trying to eat his dinner, Weber began considering the incredible possibility that something might be drastically wrong. "Three of these patients I knew very well," he says, "and there was simply no reason for them to have respiratory arrests. I took care of them day and night. I had operated on them. I literally knew them inside and out, and I knew there was no explanation for their having stopped breathing."

Perhaps choking, certainly bracing, he was beginning to suspect foul play. He'd not yet consciously thought murder, but the idea was starting to surface.

However, he wasn't going to panic, he says he decided. Everything had happened so fast, he still wanted to think. "I just kind of wanted to wait for the next day. I didn't want to get everybody excited. I thought I'd wait until the next morning and then talk to Freier and Anne Hill—I knew Anne was very interested."

At approximately 9:15 P.M. Weber was back on the hospital's front steps, getting ready to swing open one of the large entrance doors, when he suddenly heard another Code 7 called on a beeper. "I thought, 'Oh no, not again.' " The code, the sixth of the night, was on 4 East, a general surgery wing. "I went running up," he says.

Penner, too, had heard the code, and was already working on the patient when Weber arrived: "It was an old man," Penner recalls. "He had a busted hip. He had no heart rhythm and he wasn't breathing. He was even a little bit cold. So we started to work on him. He was given the bicarbonate and epinephrine. We even shocked him electrically. But he wouldn't respond. We worked on him for several minutes, but he wouldn't come back." It was to be the first death of the night.

The patient's name was Fenton Borst, sixty-five, a transfer from the Battle Creek VA hospital, who had undergone hip surgery. His condition, however, was good enough not to require intensive care. Fenton's brother Cecil, who has hired a lawyer to sue the VA, says records show that around 6 P.M. that night Fenton was checked by hospital personnel and found to be doing fine. The hospital, however, says Fenton's death was the result of a naturally occurring post-operative complication—a fat embolism, which can affect the lungs, and which sometimes occurs unexpectedly in patients undergoing bone surgery.

That is a diagnosis close to what Penner and Weber came up with. They, that night, figured Borst had suffered another kind of embolism (pulmonary). But because of Borst's proximity to what happened next, both diagnoses are questionable. For while the doctors were working frantically on Borst, one of the nurses aiding them happened to look into the room next door and discovered a seventh victim—perhaps the most suspicious arrest of the night.

"Hey, there's another one in here," Penner thinks

the nurse shouted. "When I heard that, Weber and I looked at each other like what the hell is going on?

"We ran over and here's this guy—maybe thirty-five—who looks like all he has is a broken elbow. He's got his arm in traction. I don't know his name, but he is blue! He isn't moving a muscle. And is he blue. And I was really now getting upset because this guy's a young guy. I could understand some of the older ones having an arrest, but this guy is thirty-five and all that's wrong with him is a broken elbow."

The man's name was Howard Leslie, a tall, well-built carpenter from Ypsilanti. Approximately forty (not thirty-five), Leslie had suffered a skull fracture (apparently inconspicuous by the time Penner saw him) and a broken elbow in a fall on a cement pavement while working atop a ladder. He was asleep when the arrest hit him and remembers practically nothing about the night of August 12 after approximately 8:30 P.M. when his wife left his hospital room.

"I was really worried this guy was going to die too," says Penner, "so I got very aggressive with him. He just had a little IV in a vein down here on the top of his hand. It was dripping at a very slow rate, and I was worried that the medicine wouldn't get to him fast enough. We were losing time. So while Weber was intubating him, I asked one of the medical students there for some epinephrine, and I just injected it directly into his heart. I stuck the guy right in the heart.

"It's a dangerous procedure, but by that time there were far greater risks. He had no heart rate, no breathing—no nothing. That's why I had to do something fast."

It was a good decision. After the injection, Leslie's heart rhythm started again. Later, contacted at his home, Leslie recalled coming to: "I remember someone talking to me, trying to get me to talk. But I was paralyzed. I couldn't say anything. I couldn't move my hands or feet or nothing . . . It was kind of like being dead, because you can't see anything, yet you can hear people talking." He said he knew something was strange "but I really didn't know what."

Since then Leslie has had recurring nightmares, he said, and early in 1976, he had still not been able to return to work.

But the night of the arrest, when Leslie came to, he had an endotracheal tube down his throat and was unable to talk. And although he was coming out of the coma, he was groggy, confused, and his blood pressure was low. Penner decided on another subclavian IV. He had just prepped Leslie's skin with alcohol and was preparing to insert the new needle when an eighth code was called.

"An arrest is very stressful for the patient," recalls Penner, "and I didn't want to leave him. I was worried that he might be in shock. But there was nothing I could do. I just told the nurses to keep bagging him and we'd be back as soon as we could."

The new code was back in the ICU on one of the patients who had arrested earlier—the old man with emphysema. During an intubation, resuscitators usually thrust a wooden board beneath the patient to provide resistance during chest massage. In removing this board, Penner says he was told, one of the ICU nurses had accidentally dislodged the man's endotracheal tube, and it had come out of his throat.

Both Penner and Weber felt the accident "stupid" at the least. But both say they can see how it could happen. "Those tubes are very clumsy," says Penner. "They hang over the side of the bed where they are connected to the respirator. When I got there I asked the nurse what the hell had happened, and she said it couldn't be helped. And there wasn't time to discuss it more."

Again the man had no pulse and wasn't breathing. He needed oxygen and medicine. It was another frantic resuscitation. Chest massage, injections, maybe electric shock. Complicating things was the fact that sometime during the last few codes, the resuscitations had become so fast-paced that one of the ICU nurses, it has been reported, fainted, and another suffered weak knees and nausea. Penner and Weber, consequently, were having to work all the harder.

When the doctors finally had the old man stable, it was nearing 10 P.M. Now they were able to go back to see how Leslie was doing. By this time, Leslie's own doctors were at his bedside watching his frightened eyes dart around the room. They had been summoned, probably by a call from the hospital, and they were incredulous.

Penner recalls, "They said, 'What the hell happened?' And I said, 'Well, I don't really know.' And they said, 'Well, we just can't believe it. There's no reason for him to arrest.' And they kept having me go over the details: 'What do you mean you found him blue? What do you mean he wasn't breathing?' They couldn't believe this young guy almost died, even to the point that they kept saying, 'You're positive he wasn't breathing? You're positive he didn't have a pulse?' It wasn't that they didn't trust my judgment, they were just shocked that a guy with a broken elbow could almost die."

One of Leslie's doctors finally speculated that perhaps, somehow, Leslie's apparently near-healed skull fracture had caused the arrest. There was really nothing else to blame it on. It was decided to send Leslie to the ICU where he could be better watched. The old man with emphysema still demanded attention and so

Penner had to go back to the ICU anyway. Leslie's doctors went home and Penner and Weber escorted Leslie down to the third floor.

Confident that all his patients were now out of danger, Weber says that once they reached the ICU, he, while Penner went right to work, now had a second chance to think: "I just kind of sat down and went over in my mind all that had gone on. I could understand the patient with the hip operation, but this other one [Leslie] bothered me. He confirmed my suspicions that something very strange was happening. I guess then, for the first time, I began to consciously think foul play. Somebody was putting something in the IV bottles or actually injecting it directly into the IV tubes. After going through all that, and knowing all the patients, I felt that somebody had to be doing something."

Weber, however, incredible as what he was thinking was, decided not to discuss it with anybody until he saw Freier and Hill the next morning. It was approximately midnight, he says, when things were finally calm enough that he could go home.

But Penner was still working at that time, and it wasn't until approximately 2 A.M., he recalls, that *he* finally had his chance to think.

The MOD's quarters were on the top floor of the hospital. Entering the elevator, Penner began reflecting on what he'd just gone through: "It was just like the movie *Hospital,* I thought to myself." ... Penner had seen the 1971 film ... "I had felt just like George C. Scott. Actually I'd begun to think about the movie as I was running from arrest to arrest. There were a lot of unexpected deaths in it. Someone was going around injecting patients with insulin, I believe. I'd said to one of the medical students, 'I wonder if Diana Rigg [the good-looking female lead] is going to show up?' It was just kind of a joke, but he'd said, 'Yeah, this is really weird.'"

(Penner doesn't know if the movie had recently been shown on television in Ann Arbor.)

"But as I was going up that elevator I began to think about how all the arrests had been clumped together in time and location. Like the sixth and seventh on 4 East. They were really strange. Those in the ICU you could understand. The patients were really sick. But those two—a broken hip and a broken elbow. It just didn't make sense, especially the broken elbow.

"And I had noticed that all the patients have IVs. The reason I had noticed was that when you go to an arrest one of the first things you do is put a line in the patient, an IV, because you might have to give them medicine. But each time I'd come running up I'd see that they already had an IV, and I had been grateful because it takes time to put one in. And with all these people arresting and dying, the time saved was good.

"But thinking about those IVs I suddenly got the thought that maybe there was a contaminant in the bottles. Every once in a while you hear that there's bacteria in them and people are getting infections. But then I began thinking that the facts really didn't fit that. If there was a contaminant then it was strange that the arrests were occurring to only a few patients. If there was a contaminant, arrests should be happening all over the hospital.

"IV solutions are given out at random. A guy on the third floor might get one and then a guy on the sixth floor might get the next. And they are dripped into the veins at different rates. You might get 15ccs per hour and the next guy, 5ccs. Assuming you have to reach a certain dose before the contaminant affects you, we'd have arrests all over the hospital, not just in specific places and at specific times.

"Even if the contaminant took effect with the first drop, the IVs are still hung at different times. So you'd still have the random effect. And I knew none of the arrest victims had gotten their IVs at the exact same time. I remembered as I'd run up that some of the IVs were almost full, while others were ready to be changed. The contamination idea just didn't fit. And I'm just not suspicious enough to suspect murder."

By the time he reached his room, Penner says, "I was impressed that I had just been through a bizarre sequence of events, but nothing had jelled yet." His overriding impression was exhaustion. "I knew something was weird, but I was wiped out. I just wanted to go to bed. My patients were secure and I just wanted to sleep."

But the possibility of another arrest was very real by then. And so before lying down, Penner called the hospital operator to tell her where he was and to be sure and call him if there was another. And although normally he would have taken his pocket beeper out of his pocket and deposited it on the dresser, this time he put it close to his ear. "I didn't want to miss it if it went off. That was my job, my responsibility. And you'd be surprised what you can sleep through when you're exhausted."

It was another good decision.

Penner had only been asleep about three hours when, at approximately 5:30 A.M., the beeper again suddenly went off. "I woke up and I heard someone scream, 'Oh my God, Vickers went through the window,' It was a woman's voice. It was a frantic voice."

What he probably heard was the hospital operator, whose office window might have given her a glimpse of Russell Vickers' body as it came sailing by to land on the metal grate below. Vickers, a fifty-two-year-old mental patient, had hurled himself from a fifth-floor cleaning equipment room, landing spread-eagle, smashing his skull, as well as many other bones.

Vickers' death was the first suicide at the hospital in what appears to have been almost four years. But in the next few months there would be two others. They apparently would be part of an underlying hysteria that appears to have silently gripped the hospital as the Pavulon deaths mounted and after it became known that a killer was loose in the hospital.

Vickers, an excavating contractor from a small town near Grand Rapids, had been suffering from hypertension. Patients at the hospital say he could be heard screaming on nights before his death.

"When I first woke up," says Penner. "I thought I must have been dreaming. So I rolled over. But then the phone rang and the operator said there was a code on the first floor. As I was dashing to get downstairs I was thinking, 'What could be happening on the first floor? That's where all the offices are. Maybe someone in admitting has had an arrest?' But then as I came out on the floor someone pointed outside and it hit me—Vickers went out the window!"

Penner went running outside. Vickers was lying on the grate, blood streaming from his nose and ears. He was dead. Another doctor arrived outside at about the same time, but they both pulled up short. "We both just stopped and looked at each other because we knew there wasn't anything we could do for him.

"It was a macabre sight," recalls Penner, "like something from a dark fantasy. The sun was just coming up and you could see the screen he'd knocked out, kind of dislodged in the window up above. The moon was still out and the crickets were chirping. There was a dawn shadow from the building half across his body. All that was lit was the lower part of his legs and feet. He was lying face up—his shirt open and pajama bottoms on.

Beneath the grate was a pit covering a basement window."

It was a surreal ending to an unbelievable night, and Penner, jarred by the body in front of him, was now ready to do something about it.

Chapter 7

The time of death on Vickers' death certificate is 6:05 A.M. It was probably around a half hour later that Penner went back up to the top floor to catch a little more rest. Regular hours didn't start at the hospital until 8 A.M., and by that time, he knew he'd be up, showered, and waiting at Dr. Ronald Bishop's fifth-floor office. Bishop, the head of internal medicine who at the August 4 meeting had mistaken the rising arrest rate as partly the result of a respiratory therapist shortage, was Penner's chief. "It was my job to make sure that all this came to the attention of the higher-ups," he says.

Penner's visit probably wasn't necessary. Whoever filled out the morning report for August 13—detailing what had happened the night before—had written "8 ARRESTS" in bold letters across the top of the page. It was probably one of the first things Bishop saw when he walked in. But Penner was waiting for him anyway.

Penner recalls the conversation:

"I said to him, 'What's the largest number of codes you've ever had here in a single night?' He said, 'I don't know. Why?' And I said, 'Well, there were nine last night [counting Vickers].' He just kind of exclaimed, 'Well, that's probably it. What's going on here?'"

Penner says he told the surprised Bishop about "Broken Elbow's" incomprehensible arrest, about Richards' quizzical gesturing toward his throat, about the fact that the arrests were close together in time and place and that most of the victims recovered rapidly.

"I was just throwing everything together I could, trying to find out what was going on. I may have mentioned contamination. I don't think I said murder. He [Bishop] expressed concern, but it was like he didn't know what was going on either. He was as amazed as I was."

Bishop doesn't remember much about the meeting.

"I can't recall exactly what Penner said," he relates. "He was concerned. He'd had a number of arrests the night before. But we'd had a patient who'd committed suicide. He'd jumped from a window, and we were concerned about that. That took precedent."

Bishop says a further complication was that he did not have the information needed to understand correctly what Penner was telling him.

"Most of the patients that night were surgical patients. I wasn't familiar with their cases. Penner just cited them as numbers. In general, my judgment was that this was a very unhappy occurrence but perhaps explained on the basis of their being older patients, and sick patients, and patients with respiratory disease. I guess I should have listened more closely—sat down and plotted the whole thing out and gotten a geographical distribution of things. But as I said, I was sidetracked by that suicide."

Vickers' death demanded an immediate inquiry, says Bishop. "Usually the staff and nurses are all upset. It's upsetting on the service for at least six to twelve hours.

I felt obligated to be as supportive as I could and inquire into the details to see if there wasn't something that we should have done differently to avoid or prevent it. I also was familiar with Vickers' case. I'm not sure how much I should go into his case, but I can tell you that it was the predominant thing in my mind."

When Penner, tired and shaken, left for his fourth consecutive shift (the night shift was actually two), Bishop says he temporarily put the August 12 arrests on the "back burner."

Freier, however, now nearly half a month into his acting chief of staff's job and considerably more informed, reacted differently. Press reports indicate he was soundly shocked upon opening his office and seeing the morning report.

"My God," the Detroit *Free Press* quotes him as saying to himself, "this is just unbelievable."

Since the August 4 meeting, Freier had become increasingly concerned about the mounting arrests. There were now close to forty codes recorded at the hospital since mid-July—a four-week period in which normally there would have been only about eight. The record-breaking July death figure of twenty-eight had also now been recorded, thirteen above the fifteen deaths per month which was the average for the first six months of the year.

In addition, a new statistic was beginning to loom. Under normal circumstances, a hospital usually has an arrest resuscitation rate of about 30 per cent or less. Only a relatively small number of cardiac and respiratory arrest victims are usually saved. Their bodies have to be very sick to cause the arrests in the first place. But the Ann Arbor VA, by August 12, was boasting something near a 90 per cent resuscitation rate; the hospital was reviving an amazing number of arrest victims.

Such a statistic must have come to the attention of the acting chief of staff.

So standing there that morning, probably holding the report with eight arrests detailed in it, Freier suddenly began to think the unthinkable: "It suddenly occurred to me that someone must be doing this on purpose," the Detroit *Free Press* quotes him as later telling them.

For the first time, it appears, one of the hospital's chief doctors actually became suspicious of the events of the last month or more.

Dr. Anne Hill was also close to the same conclusion by this time. It is not known exactly when she began suspecting murder, but on the morning of the twelfth she was at least discussing it.

Hill's heightened investigation, requested at the August 4 meeting, had verified her earlier finding that all the patients suffering mysterious arrests were on IVs at the time. In addition, it had revealed that all the IVs were not of the same solution. This meant that unless she had missed something, accidental contamination had to be ruled out.

Accidental contamination of a single IV solution is a conceivable rariety. But accidental contamination of several different solutions—all at the same time—is not. The solutions were produced at different places, using different materials, at different times. The odds against something going wrong with all of them simultaneously were prohibitive, probably many millions to one.

In addition, say investigators, Hill had become suspicious of some of the reactions to intubation exhibited by a few of the patients. In conversations with young residents she may have learned that the throats of supposedly natural arrest victims had accepted endotracheal tubes without the slightest problem. If this were true, then it certainly would have been alarming.

For an unanesthetized throat usually rejects the tube.

Further, although the exact date is hard to pin down, there are several reports that Hill had a nightmare about the victims around this time. The Detroit *News* quotes her as saying, "I woke up in the middle of the night and suddenly thought, 'Good God, someone is injecting muscle-paralyzing drugs into these people.'"

The paper said this was on August 15, but other reports indicate it was earlier.

Arriving at the hospital that morning, Weber, sufficiently recovered from the fatigue of the previous night, and anxious now to discuss its events, went straight to Hill's office.

He recalls: "I said, 'I'm convinced there's something wrong. I was here all night intubating and resuscitating people and there's something going on.' She said, 'Yeah, I think that's true.' As I went on, she agreed."

Discussing it awhile, the two doctors then met with Freier. Further talks ensued.

"All of us now thought something was wrong, but we didn't want to panic. We started going over the charts again trying to see if there was any common IV fluid—anything that could explain what had happened that we might have missed.

"That took all morning, but we still couldn't come up with anything. It was then that we entertained the idea of an IV purposefully contaminated—that somebody was purposefully injecting a contaminant into the IVs."

Exactly how much discussion there was of an actual murderer in their midst is not known. But it was finally decided not to call in the authorities. Weber volunteers: "I guess we still wanted to handle it ourselves ... We still hoped that somehow it would prove to be some sort of unexplainable accident."

Instead of going higher with what he knew, Freier decided more proof was needed. A formal in-house investigation would be launched. Dr. Hill was directed to draw up a memo with the circumstances of some of the most suspicious arrests. Freier was particularly taken aback, he says, by Richards' peculiar throat gesturing. "It was the classic muscle-relaxer reaction."

As the doctors dispersed, an ominous foreboding must have gone with them.

It was certainly present in the ICU.

Amid the unit's eerie wheezing noises and luminous panels, stark terror was setting in.

Lying in his open-area bed, Larry Richards was now fully awake. And his experience of the night before had frightened him considerably. He wanted to leave the ICU. He wanted to leave the hospital.

"He didn't know exactly what had happened," says his wife. "but he knew something funny was going on. He wanted out."

Although it's not clear in Mrs. Richards' mind whether her husband said the following words the day after his respiratory arrest or several days after, she remembers them vividly: "Someone's out to get me ... They [tried to] kill me once and they'll try it again."

At the time, says Mrs. Richards, she thought her husband was hallucinating. But when the news that there had been a killer in the hospital broke the following Monday, she says, she realized he hadn't been mistaken.

One of the strangest things she says her husband told her was: "They're putting laser beams in my IV."

At the time such a statement could have been (and probably was) taken as the rantings of a heavily drugged patient. But in view of what later came to light—the fact that he is an engineer—it might have been a quasi-technical description of the effects Pavulon had on his mind.

It's not likely that it was the result of an electric shock, since shocks are usually only used for heart arrests, and Richards' arrest was purely respiratory.

Several days after the thirteenth, Richards, a Korean War veteran who had sat at the Panmunjom truce talks in the early 1950s, was moved out of the ICU and into a private room on the fourth floor. His fear became so great there, says his wife, that one night after everyone had left his room he actually tried to sneak out, but was caught at the elevator.

His condition, and the fact that he had to push an IV rack along in front of him, slowed him down.

He was taken back to his room and strapped into his bed, Mrs. Richards says.

When Mrs. Richards finally learned of what had been going on in the VA, she had him moved to another hospital the very next morning.

As of early 1976, Richards was hesitant to talk even to the FBI—let alone the newspapers—his fear was still so great.

Benny Blaine, the heavy half-Chipewyan, was equally afraid, maybe more so.

By August 13, Benny was in a downhill slide that would end in his death two weeks later. The August 12 arrest, his second in three weeks, hadn't helped. His body demanded constant care. He had an incision across the entire front of his abdomen. His intestines were practically useless. A rash covered huge areas of his skin, including his groin.

(Pharmaceutical reference books say a rash sometimes breaks out on patients given Pavulon. However, many drugs cause reactions.)

A large gathering of Benny's family literally camped out at the hospital—washing him, talking to him and otherwise trying to make things easier. They would wait sometimes all day by the ICU door, or down in the VA's large front lobby. Hospital personnel still talk about them. They were allowed short, periodic visits to Benny's glass-enclosed room, most of the time in small groups.

Pete Blaine, one of Benny's adult nephews, says that around the thirteenth—the first time he'd been able to see Benny after his second arrest—one of Benny's life-support machines started "jumping" every time a certain hospital employee walked in. The name of the employee is not known because Pete, and the others who corroborate his story, never learned it. And the job of the employee, which *is* known, must, at this time, remain unstated.

But Benny's fear of the person was so great, that, through his wife, he demanded that the employee be barred from his room. A hospital official who was there later confirmed that the employee was asked to comply with Benny's wishes, but only because the hospital didn't want him agitated. In reality, they only believed he was unduly paranoid.

After the family was assured that the employee would be kept out, however, Pete says he overheard Benny tell his [Benny's] wife, Cora, "[the employee] is the one giving me the shots ... the one making me sick." Cora confirms that Benny made the charges, and Benny's married sisters, Betty and Delsie, say they heard Benny say approximately the same thing.

"My uncle couldn't read or write," says Pete, a shipping and receiving foreman, "but he wasn't stupid. He knew something was happening to him. The hospital told my aunt he was hallucinating, that he didn't know what he was saying. But my uncle was afraid. He wouldn't let [the employee] touch him or get near him."

One hospital official, however, says all this occurred *after* it became public knowledge there was a killer in the VA.

By late afternoon August 13, Dr. Hill had completed her memo and turned it in to Freier. Included in the list of arrests that the red-haired anesthesiologist was concerned about, according to Freier, were the names of Lutz, Stout, Blaine and Richards—perhaps a dozen in all.

Hill also made a recommendation: "I'd like to ask that we have an inquiry into these sudden arrests," the memo is quoted as saying. "I've collected what information I can, but I'd suggest a panel to talk to the physician on the spot in all cases. In both last night's and the previous run of arrests, the only common factor I can come up with is they mostly occur at night and most [of the patients] have IVs running.

"I have studied as many charts as possible but need more assistance. I feel the people on the spot—both nurses and physicians—could give valuable information that might yield the answer, if there is one. We have a quiet schedule tomorrow. If interviews could be started then, it would be best. Here's a list of some, but not all, of the arrest victims."

The familiar names then followed.

According to a variety of reports, Hill's recommendation was adopted. A panel was selected. A member of the lay administration staff was even assigned to serve on it.

But even before the panel began its deliberations, the killer, or killers, subsequent events would prove, was readying to strike again. And when the hospital, two days later, finally would be forced to call in the FBI, six more patients—probably the most that had ever died there in a similar period—would be dead.

It was probably late when Freier, Weber and Hill left the hospital for their homes on August 13. Night, now feared by the entire hospital, had already begun to fall.

Chapter 8

Thunderstorms and a low of 60 degrees were predicted for Ann Arbor the night of August 14. Dr. Joe Zibrak, black-haired Ann Arbor VA intern from New York City, however, was unaware of the cooling weather. Trying to control a berserk mental patient in the hospital's basement, things were hot for him.

It was about 9 or 9:15 P.M. when Zibrak, MOD that night, had been summoned from the fifth floor where he'd been attending patients. The berserk veteran, young and big, had been attempting to sign out of the hospital against medical advice when he'd started having uncontrollable seizures. Most of the hospital supervisory personnel on that night were down in the basement trying to find out what was happening. In addition to doctors, there were nurses, hospital security guards, even some administrative people. No one could get close enough to the patient to inject Valium, a tranquilizer; every time someone approached, he'd start swinging. Backed up against the basement's beige tile walls, the patient was in a highly defensible position.

Nobody in the basement knew it at the time, but it is now believed that the unintentional bottom-floor commotion probably allowed the Ann Arbor VA killer (or killers) to roam and kill at will. In the next two hours, five patients would arrest, three of them would die and one of the victims would go into a coma from which he would never emerge and in which he would die approximately two weeks later.

All of the five victims would eventually be placed high on official lists of suspected Pavulon attacks.

In retrospect, the night of August 14 would become one of the most chilling in the entire Ann Arbor investigation. For if the basement diversion really did provide the killer (or killers) with a chance to roam freely, then the patients attacked probably experienced all the horrors that can possibly be associated with a Pavulon injection.

Several of the victims were in private, out-of-the-way rooms, and thus their lives, silently but tortuously slipping from them, were entirely dependent on a chance discovery by bed-checking personnel. Paralyzed, they couldn't have called out.

In addition, most of the victims appear to have been conscious at the time of their attacks, conscious and alert. Thus they probably fully felt the fear and claustrophobic panic that would have accompanied the slow suffocation.

The thought of such deaths must play heavily on the minds of the hospital staff as the case goes to trial. But on the night of August 14, Zibrak and the others in the basement were wholly occupied with the rampaging patient. Zibrak was aware of the high number of arrests at the hospital, but they hadn't made that big an impression on him yet.

"I'd worked in larger hospitals than the VA during my training," he says, "and there weren't as many arrests. But I attributed the high number to the fact that the VA has a lot of sick patients. A VA is really a cross between a nursing home and an acute care hospital. A lot of patients come here in the terminal stages of their illnesses. The families can no longer bear the emotional and economic expense. And there's no motivation to get them out because the government's paying.

"I thought having arrests was the normal state of affairs at the VA," he says.

Assisting Zibrak in the basement were Dr. Mike Mcleod, SOD (surgeon of the day) and also an intern, and Dr. Bob Wise, a second-year resident (called a house officer III) in internal medicine.

Mcleod, a twenty-five-year-old Cornell graduate from New York, also knew about the high number of arrests. But like Zibrak, he felt they were the result of the VA's high proportion of very sick patients—even more so. He had heard about August 12 from Weber, his surgical superior. The nine codes were the "talk of the hospital," according to its younger doctors. "But I thought everyone was getting unduly alarmed," says Mcleod. "You might say I'm naive. I just couldn't conceive that anything could really be wrong."

Wise, older than Zibrak and Mcleod, says he knew "something crazy was going on," but his ideas about it had not progressed beyond the "grim humor" stage—"the only way we could deal with it in those days."

Wise, however, was seriously perplexed over at least one patient. Robert Antil, the forty-one-year-old Detroit steelworker mentioned earlier in relation to Emmett Lutz's July 26 arrest, had probably suffered more arrests than any other patient during July and August—some say as many as fourteen, although six or seven appears more correct. Wise was perplexed because in most of the cases, Antil exhibited the same unusual pattern: he'd be doing fine, says Wise, then he'd suddenly arrest and be easily resuscitated. There was seldom, if ever, any clinical reason for the arrests.

(It's not clear how many of the arrests were respiratory, but the number, according to those familiar with his case, was substantial.)

Antil had heart problems and was in the last stages of diabetes. But, says Wise, "in retrospect, he had a fairly typical pattern for a Pavulon death."

It took a long time—over an hour, according to Zibrak—but a group of those down in the basement finally subdued the berserk patient. Zibrak was on top of him trying to insert an IV in his arm, he says, when he got the first page.

"It said simply that a doctor was needed on 5 East," he recalls. "I couldn't go because I was sitting on top of this guy. So I asked somebody to find out what the page was about. They came back and gave me the message that it was not an emergency and would I please call back when I got a chance."

It appears that by that time two patients upstairs had already died. The page, Zibrak eventually learned, was for him, MOD, to come up and formally pronounce Roy Ogle and James Oulds dead. The two patients neither of them acutely ill, had been found dead in their beds. There never was a chance of resuscitation. No codes were even called.

Ogle, fifty-seven, of Ann Arbor, was a chronic alcoholic. He'd been treated periodically at the VA for alcoholism. Earlier in the day on August 14, according to an official written report about his case, he'd come to the VA and told the admitting doctor that he'd consumed between "five and seven fifths of wine" the night before, and had eaten little in the past two weeks. In admitting him, the VA doctor had listed "early alcohol abstinence syndrome" as the diagnosis, and started him on an IV of nourishment and tranquilizers.

All that was really wrong with Ogle, according to the report, was that he had the shakes and might go into the DTs—rarely a fatal complication.

He was put on 5 East, a general medicine floor.

Oulds, sixty-three, was a retired coal miner living in Flint, Michigan, and the only Negro suspected of having been attacked at the hospital. Not much is publicly known about Oulds. Not only does the hospital—as it does with all suspected victims—refuse to talk about him, but his family in Flint has also turned down requests for interviews. But records show that Oulds suffered from kidney failure, and, according to one doctor familiar with his case, he was in the hospital the day he died solely for a periodic hemodialysis, a machine cleansing of his blood.

His death certificate, however, says he also had blood infection and a chronic lung condition caused by dust from the coal mines.

He, too, had been assigned a bed on 5 East—right across from Ogle's.

Apparently the berserk patient in the basement was still putting up a fight, for Zibrak had not yet been able to get the tranquilizer into him when he received a second page. This time the message was more detailed: two persons had died and the nurses wanted him to come up and pronounce the men dead.

"My response was shock," says Zibrak. "No one had told me any of our medicine patients [on 5 East] were critically ill. And as a matter of fact the two people who died had only been admitted that day, and neither of them, especially Mr. Ogle, was thought to have been anywhere near dying."

Suddenly the berserk patient didn't pose such a problem anymore. "We got things under control rather rapidly," recalls Zibrak. Wise and he took the patient back up to the psychiatric ward and strapped him into bed. At approximately 10:45 P.M., with the two doctors studying the young veteran's chart and hoping to talk to the nurses soon about what had happened to Ogle and Oulds, the first code of the evening was called.

The arrest was in the coronary care unit, a large, enclosed room off to the right of the ICU entrance. It usually held four heart patients.

The patient having the arrest was named James Hall. Little is publicly known about Hall. (It has not been mentioned yet, but doctors oftentimes felt ethically bound not to use a patient's name when discussing him with someone other than family or friends. For this reason, as well as others, identities of certain arrest victims were never learned. Subsequent personal information about them was also missed.)

One investigator says Hall might have yelled for help. But that has never been verified. The first doctor at Hall's bedside was Mcleod. After the basement patient had been subdued, Mcleod had gone to 4 West, a surgical ward, where many of his patients were. Being closest to the ICU, he was the first to arrive.

"He [Hall] was out when I got there," recalls Mcleod. "I remember attempting to intubate him. But I didn't have the proper stylet [a wire support used to give maneuverability to the soft endotracheal tube], and a nurse had to get me another." Zibrak and Wise soon arrived. "I remember Wise bagging the patient."

Hall was in the ICU because it was feared he might have a heart attack. But there is confusion over whether his heart was working normally when the doctors began the intubation. Mcleod says he thinks Hall had no heart rhythm, but "the details are very vague and I wouldn't emphasize anything." Zibrak, however, says Hall did have a pulse (meaning an effective heart rhythm). "It was primarily that he wasn't breathing."

Whatever the truth, when the murders were finally discovered and doctors reexamined all the suspicious arrests, they listed Hall as having one of the ten most suspicious." It seems unlikely that they would have done that had they been able to blame the arrest on his heart.

In addition, says Zibrak, Hall came out of the arrest very easily, an indication to some that it was not a cardiac arrest or heart malfunction. The three doctors had not been attending to Hall more than a few minutes when a second code was called.

The suspicious pattern of arrests in quick succession was unfolding again.

The second code was back on the fifth floor—where Ogle and Oulds had died—but at the other end, on 5 West.

Joseph Green, seventy-eight, a retired insurance salesman from Parchment, Michigan, outside Kalamazoo, had checked into the hospital in late July with an infection around his implanted pacemaker, a small, matchbox-sized machine that stimulates heart contractions electrically. Heart disease had disrupted Green's natural stimulus, and the pacemaker had been implanted just below his left collarbone. But in 1974, pus began to form around the apparatus, and after surgery to replace it, a further infection developed along the pacemaker wire extending into his heart.

As explained by his wife, the wire traveled up under the skin to the collarbone, where it entered a main vein through which it then went back down to one of the heart's large chambers. However, the new infection had caused the wire to break through the skin in places and erupted lengths of it could actually be seen on Green's chest. Doctors determined that the wire had to be removed, but it couldn't simply be pulled out. During the long period it had been inside Green, the wire had become embedded in the vein's walls—probably the reason it hadn't been removed when the old pacemaker had been replaced. It was stuck, and on August 14 Green was in a private room awaiting the necessary surgery, scheduled for the following day.

He was in pain, but not in any immediate danger, according to his wife.

Pictures Mrs. Green has of her husband show a short, stocky man with a pleasant smile. He had been a baker in the Navy during World War I. Their son (they also have a daughter) is an Army officer. August 14 Mrs. Green spent the entire day with her husband, she relates. He was fine. At about 8:30 P.M., she says, someone came to the room to take blood. The person was with her husband about a half hour. Then he was taken down for X rays. When he returned, he was "sleepy," she says, and at about 9:15 P.M. she decided to leave.

That was the last time she saw him alive. "It was so unexpected," she says over and over.

Green was discovered, it appears, sometime around 10:45 P.M.—approximately an hour and a half after Mrs. Green left. A nurse found him, says Zibrak. Once Zibrak heard the code, it probably took him several moments to get up to the fifth floor. Mcleod, who stayed with Hall, arrived a short time later.

When he arrived, with one med student accompanying him, Zibrak says that Green was "totally out." He had no heartbeat and wasn't breathing. There was no telling how long he'd been that way, says Zibrak, and he immediately began cardiac massage while at the same time instructing that an "ambu" bag be placed over Green's mouth in an attempt to force air into his lungs.

Mcleod was the first to try and intubate Green, but, he says, he found Green's vocal cords in "severe spasm." "Laryngeal edema," another complication, had also set in. The cords were swollen and contracted. He couldn't get the endotracheal tube past them.

Zibrak tried, but he too couldn't loosen the cords.

The problem was crucial, the two doctors realized, for it they couldn't get Green's airway open, there would be no way of reviving his heart.

They resumed resuscitation efforts all the harder, Mcleod working on getting the tube down Green's throat and Zibrak on his heart.

A few moments of feverish effort passed. Then one of the nurses assisting the resuscitators said that a patient across the hall was lying abnormally still. His head was at a curious angle. Going over to check on him she discovered that he too was in arrest.

No code was called. Resuscitators were already on the floor. Zibrak ran to the patient's bedside. His name was Adam Oelberg, a fifty-nine-year-old California forest worker from Saginaw.

Oelberg's gray-blue eyes were open and staring, but Zibrak quickly realized he wasn't seeing anything out of them.

He was pulseless and breathless.

Mcleod too, as soon as he got a chance, rushed over to see if he was needed. But Zibrak said he felt he could handle it himself.

Until only a few years before, Oelberg, 5'7", 160 pounds, according to a California driver's license issued him in 1971, was a vigorous outdoorsman working for the Inglewood, California, Parks Department. The license shows him with a white walrus mustache. Coming from Russian immigrant parents, says his sister in Saginaw, he loved music and often played a hand accordion at German-American dances. But then, she says, diabetes began to debilitate him. He lost several of his toes (they had to be amputated because the tissue had died), suffered increasing pain when walking and eventually became hospitalized. A family member had gone out to California at the beginning of the year to bring him back home.

Since then Oelberg had lost the sight in one eye and had developed a mysterious pain in his hip. He'd first been in the Saginaw VA hospital, and had recently been transferred to Ann Arbor for exploratory surgery. Like Green, he was scheduled for the operating table the following day when he was discovered in arrest.

Zibrak went frantically to work. He pounded on Oelberg's chest. He had someone bag him. He gave him medicine. Intermittently he ran back to Green's bedside to see what he could do there. As soon as he could, he put a tube down Oelberg's throat and started him breathing mechanically. Powerful electric shocks were administered for his heart. Eventually Oelberg's vital signs improved. He began coming back.

Green, however, continued to remain the same.

Mcleod and the others tried every procedure possible, but Green just wouldn't respond.

He was turning bluer by the minute.

For a while, Mcleod had mistaken a false heartbeat generated by Green's pacemaker as a sign that perhaps he might be rallying. He had increased his efforts all the more. But the false hope had quickly been realized for what it was.

It appears there never really was any chance to save Green. He had been too far gone by the time the doctors had reached him.

It is not clear exactly when the following occurred, but after Hall downstairs was stabilized, Wise, who had stayed behind to work on him, was finally able to come up to 5 West and lend another pair of hands. In a last-ditch measure, Wise and Mcleod performed a tracheotomy on Green—an emergency operation in which a hole is cut into the patient's throat in hopes of getting air into his lungs. But the effort was useless.

"His pupils were dilated and he was totally unresponsive," recalls Mcleod. "That's usually an indication that the brain is gone and the patient is irretrievable."

Seeing that there was nothing more they could do for Green, the intubators gave up.

They had worked nearly half an hour on the patient, they say.

Eventually, Oelberg was brought back to a near-vegetable state. But he never would come out of the coma. He would die eleven days later, on August 25.

It wasn't until past midnight that the three young doctors finally got a chance to reflect on what had happened: three dead, one dying, a fifth just missing death. Each of the doctors had been involved in frantic resuscitations before, but nothing like this. Strangely, however, they still didn't suspect murder. It was still, for most, inconceivable. Also, as the arrests became more commonplace at the hospital, they also became, ironically, more acceptable, more "normal" to the young doctors. They, unlike their superiors, didn't have the advantage of the big picture.

Still, they tried hard to come up with an explanation. Contamination was mentioned. In the case of Green, according to Wise, it was even speculated that perhaps some kind of freak electrical accident had occurred involving, perhaps, his pacemaker. An electrocution? It was hard to comprehend, but such things could happen in a hospital, especially in view of the metal frames on most hospital beds. And, "Well," says Wise, "it entered our minds."

When the shift finally ended, each was deeply affected. Perhaps, if they had had more time, they might have eventually settled on what, in retrospect, seems obvious: a deranged murderer (or murderers) was taking advantage of every concealed moment to kill, terrorize and maim.

But they didn't have more time.

The attacks were now the result of a seemingly new and bolder onslaught. The killer (or killers) was becoming more brazen every day. And before the young doctors would have a chance to sit down and coolly dissect what had happened, almost the entire hospital would be shocked into the murder realization by a series of daylight attacks committed practically in front of everyone already concerned with the arrests that July and early August.

Chapter 9

It was Friday, August 15, approximately 4:30 P.M. The ICU was packed. All the beds were full. Doctors, nurses, orderlies—maybe even visitors—walked back and forth. Shifts had just changed. Most were either starting things up or winding them down. Among those present were Penner and Weber, who had answered the eight codes August 12; Bishop, Penner's superior, trying to make room for a drug overdose patient just admitted; and Mcleod, the surgical intern, who along with Zibrak had fought the deadly arrests the night before.

Outside it was drizzling.

Mcleod was attending a patient. Suddenly a nurse called out to him—presumably because he was the closest doctor to her—that Benny Blaine, the heavy half-Chipewyan recovering from abdominal surgery, was having trouble. Blaine was still in one of the glass-enclosed private rooms. Although he was newly infused with a fear that someone was trying to make him "sick," he had rallied from his August 12 arrest, and doctors were thinking of moving him out of the ICU to accommodate the drug overdose.

Now, however, he wasn't looking so good.

Mcleod, and possibly another surgeon nearby, went over.

"I went in and asked him what was the matter," Mcleod says. "He just shrugged like he didn't know. He couldn't speak. But he was gradually becoming weak and blue. He just gestured like he didn't know what was happening. Apparently he couldn't take the deep breaths needed to maintain his oxygenation, and so his hemoglobin was being reduced. Blue is the color of reduced hemoglobin."

According to several witnesses, Blaine's heart monitor showed normal activity. He was not experiencing a cardiac arrest. And approximately thirty seconds after Mcleod entered the room, he says, Blaine went limp. (Others there have termed the condition "flaccid.") It was then, Mcleod says, that he decided Blaine needed to be resuscitated, and grabbing an "ambu" bag, he sounded the alarm.

The unexpected arrest—now officially believed to be the result of a Pavulon attack (although unrealized at that moment) in broad daylight—must have immediately attracted the attention of practically everyone in the ICU. People came running from all directions. Weber, one of the senior residents present, began the intubation. Bishop—for the first time witnessing one of the suspicious arrests (although he might not have suspected its criminal nature at that precise time) —handed implements. Others, like Penner, quickly formed a group of anxious onlookers that spilled out of Blaine's room and into the adjacent hallway.

Not everyone could take part in the resuscitation.

One of the last doctors to arrive at the arrest was Lucy Goodenday, chief of cardiology, until now not involved in the arrests.

Thirty-eight, New York-born and -schooled, Dr.

Goodenday had joined the VA staff in late June, only six weeks before. Her last hospital position had been in San Francisco. The job of cardiology chief had been a step up in her career. She was now one of the permanent VA staff members, along with Freier, Bishop and Hill.

Dr. Goodenday, she says, had been on the eighth floor when Blaine's code had been called. Cardiologists are always needed at arrests, so she'd rushed down. But by the time she'd arrived there were already more than enough doctors. She'd joined the others watching from the periphery.

On the same floor was the coronary care unit, or CCU, a larger room where the acute heart patients— all of them, ultimately, under Dr. Goodenday's supervision—were kept. During Blaine's arrest, the CCU's door was open, and concerned that some of the cardiac patients might get overly excited from all the commotion, Dr. Goodenday says she began periodically checking to see that they were all right.

Suddenly, during one of her checks, she says, she noticed a CCU patient in a corner bed on the far side of the room looking "agitated." There was a nurse standing by him, she says, and she went in to see what was the matter. When she reached the bedside—probably no more than thirty to forty feet away—she says, the patient was "struggling to tell us something, but obviously he couldn't. He couldn't talk."

The patient's name was John McCrery, a forty-nine-year-old Coloma, Michigan, auto body shop owner-operator, who had been admitted to the VA on August 4 with chest pains and an irregular heartbeat. Although on the surface he seemed to be doing reasonably well, McCrery was considered dangerously close to a heart attack, and was scheduled for open-heart surgery in the next few days.

Naturally Dr. Goodenday was concerned about him. But after she got to his bedside, it didn't appear that his heart was the problem.

"I asked him, 'Are you having any chest pain?' He shook his head no. I asked if he was having trouble breathing. He nodded yes. I asked him to take a deep breath, but he couldn't. Initially he could move a little. But very rapidly he couldn't do anything. Then, within seconds, everything just seemed to stop."

McCrery, others would verify, went flaccid.

This was the first of the suspicious arrests that Goodenday had witnessed. As a staff member, she had been aware of the arrest problem at the hospital, but until this very moment—as she stood there observing McCrery's strange behavior—she says she had not become overly alarmed about it. Now, seeing one of the arrests with her own eyes, she became troubled. She couldn't understand what was happening.

But at that precise instant there wasn't time to contemplate. She yelled "Arrest," and at the same time moved to the head of the bed to begin clearing McCrery's airway.

By this time, it appears, Blaine, across the hall, was stabilized and on a respirator. Perhaps ten minutes had elapsed since the first code had been called. Weber, Bishop and the others rushed over. An attempt to put a tube down McCrery's throat was made. But the tube was too big, says Goodenday. Looking out in the hallway, Goodenday spied Anne Hill, generally regarded as one of the best intubators in the hospital at that time. She called for the anesthesiologist's help. Hill rushed in.

Hill, it has been reported, had, like Goodenday, arrived after the first code had sounded, but a bit later. In one of the few interviews she gave, she told the Associated Press that she had been on the fourth floor preparing to hold a meeting when one of her doctors received word of Blaine's arrest. "We always respond," she told the interviewer. So grabbing her resuscitation kit, says the story, she hurried down.

When she arrived, wrote the AP reporter, Blaine was already on an artificial respirator and "everything was under control. Then she heard the call from the coronary care unit [and] dashed across the hall."

Hill set right to work, says Goodenday. But she too encountered trouble. McCrery's throat and the oversized intubation tube were the main problems, according to accounts. Reluctantly but skillfully, accounts indicate, she forced the larger tube in.

Meanwhile—probably to the astonishment of practically everyone there—a third code was called. It was in the other glass-enclosed private room in the ICU. (Both small rooms were right together.) The patient was William Loesch, the young Vietnam veteran with the gunshot wound. Loesch, like Blaine, had last suffered what is believed to have been an attack on August 12. Now, like Blaine, he was in arrest again. (It was the third believed attack for both.)

Dr. Ira "Jeff" Strumpf, a senior medicine resident from Miami, Florida, was the first physician known to have observed Loesch in trouble that day.

"I was standing in the hall watching [the McCrery resuscitation]," he recalls. "Someone—I can't remember who—called me into his [Loesch's] room. He was lying prone and ... conscious ... but it looked like he was having trouble breathing.

"At first I thought it was just a hysteria thing. I ordered him to breathe. But he couldn't. He just moved his lips trying to say, 'I can't breathe.' In retrospect I see it was probably Pavulon because it overtook him so fast. But for a moment there, I didn't think it was real."

(This was the time that Loesch subsequently told the Detroit *Free Press* reporter "I felt a pain in my IV. I rolled over ..." Then, within half a minute, he lost control of his eyes. "My whole body felt like it went up in flames, and that was it.")

Seeing Loesch try to mouth the words, Strumpf says he realized the young veteran "wasn't kidding."

Nearby was a respiratory therapist whom Strumpf knew and had confidence in, he says. He ran outside the room, he says, presumably gave the alarm and asked the therapist to aid him. Shortly thereafter, Weber and some others came running over and the third intubation began full scale.

Back in the CCU, McCrery was now on a respirator, limp and seemingly unresponsive. Unknown to the two women physicians working over him, however, was the fact that although he appeared to be unconscious, he actually could hear and feel.

In fact, he says, he was cognizant of everything from the beginning.

"What happened," said McCrery, in an interview two and a half months after the incident, "was that I got what I thought was medication. But it turned out to be a paralyzer of some sort."

It was a nurse who had given him the shot, he said.

At home and recuperating, he could talk easily about it.

"It was put in the IV tube, which is a common thing. I mean most of our medication came through the IV. So, at the time I got the shot, I didn't think anything of it."

But within ten to fifteen seconds, he says, he knew something was wrong. "I didn't know what, but I was practically paralyzed.

"It was a feeling of general numbness," he says. When he realized something was wrong, he says, he turned to find the nurse who had injected it into his IV walking away.

He tried to call out for help but got no response.

It was probably just prior to this point that Dr. Goodenday noticed him "agitated," and walked in.

Helplessness quickly overtook him, says McCrery. "The first thing I lost was my voice, because I tried to say something to the nurse walking away, but nothing would come out. All I could do was gesture. I think my vision was the last to go. I don't remember if I saw Dr. Goodenday come in, or just could hear her. But I remember her talking to me."

Goodenday had given McCrery some tests, he says, and had consulted with him several times about his upcoming operation. He knew her voice.

"I remember her asking if I was okay—could I say anything to her? Maybe my eyes were open for a while. Maybe she thought she could get through to me. I don't know. All I can remember is that I wanted to answer her. Oh yes I did! But I couldn't. And apparently I stopped breathing about that time, because she sounded the alarm."

The next thing that stands out in his memory was a jolt.

"When it's an emergency, they really hustle. I had the sensation of being thrown back on a flat board like a piece of plywood or something. I could feel my head snap back—which they have to do apparently—and I still have the sensation of them pounding on my chest. I thought they were going to break my ribs. I imagine they were trying to get me to breathe. They really beat you."

McCrery's monitor showed erratic heart activity during the arrest, says Goodenday. But there's no question, she adds, that the aberration was an "effect" of his breathing stoppage, not a "cause."

The chest pounding, then, was probably a reaction to the aberration, which had followed the breathing stoppage.

It wasn't very long, says McCrery, before he recognized the voice of another doctor—the Irish brogue of Anne Hill.

"Apparently she must have been close by. Because it didn't seem very long until she was there. She was quite active in the [resuscitation]. I could hear her saying 'get me this' and 'get me that.' That's when they were going to put a tube down my throat to hook me up to the breathing machine.

"I think she said she wanted a No. 2 size tube. Now I don't know anything about those tubes, but I assume there are different tubes for different people. But the one she wanted wasn't available and she was very upset. She said something to the effect of 'With all the respiratory arrests that have been taking place they certainly should have what they need on the emergency cart.' She was quite perturbed."

(It's possible that the multiple arrests in the ICU temporarily depleted an adequate supply of resuscitation equipment. It's also possible that the cart was deliberately sabotaged. Unconfirmed reports, not necessarily about the August 15 arrests, have alleged just that.)

Someone was sent out to find a smaller tube, says McCrery, "but apparently they didn't have one." The next thing he remembers, he says, is Hill saying, "This man's throat is going to be sore for six weeks." Then, after a period of silence, he says he heard, "Okay, it's down." After he'd been hooked up to the respirator, he remembers: "It's working . . . We've got him on it."

Strangely, McCrery doesn't recall any feeling of suffocation.

"I didn't feel a sensation of choking. The feeling was

discomforting—more like being hypnotized or paralyzed. Yes, paralyzed. That's exactly what it felt like ... But I didn't have the feeling of wanting air, like when you hold your breath."

Apparently the intubation was performed that quickly.

When Hill had first rushed into the CCU, says Goodenday, she had asked the cardiologist, "Did you see it?" Goodenday, almost astonished at her own words, had answered, "Yes. It looked like ... like curare?"

Later that afternoon she would recall that a friend had once written a science fiction story in which the jungle poison and its paralyzing action had played a part.

"I'd never been to South America—never even used the medication—but it was the only thing I could think of."

Apparently the outward manifestations of McCrery's arrest—the suddenness of it, the apparent total paralysis—were enough to make the cardiologist instantly suspect muscle relaxer.

Hill, all available evidence suggests, had already been considering it.

For example, the theory that murder was responsible for the hospital's high arrest rate had, by August 15, been tagged the "Hill-Freier syndrome."

By this time, Freier, who, he says, had come into the ICU during Loesch's resuscitation, had joined Goodenday and Hill. Bishop, still faced with solving the problem posed by the drug overdose patient, had gone upstairs to look for more beds.

Freier, too, was thinking muscle relaxer. "We suddenly realized all three were very flaccid," he later told the *Medical World News*.

Now the three medical chiefs needed to know exactly which type of muscle relaxer they were faced with. Different types require different antidotes.

Hill, say the other two, suggested a nerve stimulation test.

An anesthesiologist should know about muscle relaxers and their control. The stimulation test would show them whether the victims had been injected with a curare-like relaxer or a relaxer from one of the other groups.

Relaxers work by disrupting the chemical communication between nerve endings and muscle receptors. The nerve stimulator, a hand-held device, bridges the disruption with an electrical current. The muscles react artificially.

Depending on the specific reaction of the patient, the tester can tell which relaxer group is present.

What happened next is still hazy. But the following is an approximation from varying accounts.

Hill went to get a stimulator. She had to go to the fourth floor to get it. It took her between five and ten minutes.

When she returned, it was approximately 5:30 P.M.—about one hour since the arrests had begun. McCrery was lying seemingly lifeless on his bed, a mask from the respirator covering his mouth.

She went quickly to work. Two wires from the stimulator, which can be either battery- or socket-powered, were inserted into McCrery's forearm. The current was switched on. Nothing happened. One witness thinks the wires may have been inadequately placed.

Hill tried again. This time the wires were inserted in a different manner. The power was again turned on. Suddenly McCrery's hand moved. It curled in the specific way that indicated the test was yielding positive results.

McCrery recalls: "I could hear some talk about finding out what kind of drug I was on ... They weren't sure what it was ... Apparently there are two or three or four that could do it and they didn't know for sure.

"So all of a sudden, in my left arm, I could feel ... well, it was like a shock or poking sensation or something. And I heard them talking. And I think it was Dr. Hill that asked me, 'Can you hear us?' ... And I could hear them and I could feel it in my arm ... But I couldn't respond."

Not knowing McCrery's thoughts, Hill grabbed his curling hand and began feeling intensely. She was searching for a certain inner "twitching" that could only be felt within the tissues. It would be another sign that what they suspected was correct. Only a trained physician could detect it.

She found the twitching. There probably was some sort of audible confirmation. The test was positive. It was certain now. They'd found the relaxer group. It was, as they had first surmised, the curare group, one of which was pancuronium, the generic name of the trade relaxer Pavulon.

Pavulon was the main relaxer the hospital stocked. In fact, at least one patient in the ICU was actually on the drug.

It was around and available.

"Everyone just had an amazed look on their faces," says Goodenday.

Now they needed an antidote.

"I asked Anne if she knew anything that would reverse it," says Goodenday. "She said yes."

What Hill came up with was neostigmine, an antidote for various muscle dysfunctions, possibly mixed with atropine, a drug to counteract unwanted side effects.

Neostigmine worked on some of the curare synthetics, but not all. Some were irreversible.

Tension must have risen.

Across the hall, Blaine, in the private room, had been resuscitated. But he too was seemingly unresponsive. His large body heaved with the respirator. Because neostigmine was particularly prone to cause problems in heart patients, it was decided to try the antidote on him first since his heart was fine.

Holding an ampule of the reversing agent, Hill moved across to Blaine's room. "I hoped I was wrong," the AP story quoting her says she thought to herself. "But if the antidote worked it meant her worst suspicions were true—that someone was running around the hospital paralyzing patients, and that [that] someone was probably not too distant."

Before she injected the antidote, says the AP, she asked Blaine, "Open your eyes. Squeeze my hand. Lift your head. Take a deep breath." Apparently the questions were actually commands. He could do none of those things, but she hoped that shortly he could.

She inserted the syringe's tip into Blaine's IV— the same place that it is believed the killer used when injecting the Pavulon—and squeezed. Not more than a moment or two passed before the patient started to react. Blaine's eyes opened, says the AP. He squeezed her hand.

It was a "classical" reversal, says Goodenday. "He came out of it almost immediately."

There were probably shouts of jubilation. They had the right reversing agent. In addition, they had concrete proof of what they were up against, and they now knew how to handle it.

But no one took much time to reflect on the success. There were two other patients to be reversed, and the thought might have occurred to some of those present that maybe the others had been given different relaxers. The probability was not great, but apprehension probably returned.

The group now moved to McCrery. (It is certain that atropine was added to McCrery's antidote.)

McCrery remembers: "For a while, I thought I was dead. You know, you get that crazy feeling. You think maybe I'm dead but I'm not completely dead. I can hear them [and feel the nerve stimulator test] but I'm gone.

"But then I could hear them talking again and they said, 'Well, let's try the antidote.' "

Shortly, he says, he felt another electric shock— "like I'd grabbed a live wire or something ... It felt like it went all through my entire body."

Following the antidote, says Goodenday, Hill gave McCrery a second nerve-stimulation test to verify that the antidote was working.

"All of a sudden," says McCrery, "either I opened my eyes, or moved my hand or something, because then I heard Dr. Hill say: 'Look at that! Look at that! He's responding! Look at that.'

"She was so enthused. And I knew it was her. I still couldn't see. It was too sudden. But I felt a whole lot better. I said, 'Well, I guess I'm not dead.' Because it had been in my mind that I must be dead. You can't really phrase how you felt.

"But Dr. Hill was enthused with my response—and apparently not only for my sake. But also because they'd finally pinpointed what was going on so they'd know what to do from then on if they had another arrest."

It was a turning point. Hill and Freier, at least, now believed that their worst fears had been realized: there was a killer among them.

They must have moved guardedly to the third victim's room.

Chapter 10

When Dr. Goodenday first observed McCrery, her initial thought had been contamination. "Perhaps a drug had been mislabeled," she says she surmised. "Perhaps he got someone else's drug order. The idea of a purposeful contamination was too farfetched. Muscle relaxers weren't poisons. If used properly, there wasn't any danger."

But now after watching the reversals and having had a chance to think about it all, she was having second thoughts. She didn't have the benefit of the close study of the past month's arrests as did Freier and Hill. Now she wondered, could it be that this wasn't an accident? That somebody had actually purposefully caused the arrests?

The questions were, to say the least, alarming. And suddenly she realized she was fearful.

When the others left McCrery's room for Loesch's, she stayed behind. She and McCrery were now alone. His eyes were anxious. The intubation tube bulged in his mouth. His throat was probably hurting. Muffled coughs might have been sounding through the respirator.

She approached him.

"He had a tube in place and couldn't talk," she recalls. "I asked him 'Did you remember everything that had gone on?' He nodded yes. 'Were you conscious?' He nodded yes.

"He was very animated and vociferous. It appeared he was trying to tell me something. I asked him, 'Did you receive any medication immediately before the arrest had occurred?' He nodded yes.

" 'Did you see who?' "

Again he nodded yes.

The cardiologist now wanted more.

"I gave him a piece of paper," she says, "and he wrote down a name."

What exactly was on the note, Goodenday would not then reveal. But she confirmed later that it was a nickname—"a strange nickname"—and that eventually it was linked to a nurse.

McCrery says he doesn't remember giving the note to Goodenday. But he confirms that the FBI has shown him one with a nickname on it, and because they have told him he wrote it, he says he feels he probably did.

But he says his mind is clear about what happened to him just prior to the arrest. Although he too is reluctant to give specifics, he confirms that the person he saw near his bedside was a nurse and that he'd know her if he saw her again.

Here, in essence, is what he said about the nurse in a taped interview November 1, 1975:

He had been moved just that morning into the corner bed he occupied when he suffered the late afternoon arrest. It was close to the CCU's window, and had been vacated when Mark Hogan, the elderly heart patient who had experienced some fully conscious arrests in July and early August, had died around 8 A.M.

Hogan's son had given him a *Reader's Digest,* and he'd been alternately leafing through it and dozing since early afternoon. "They had me on so much medication I was usually tired.

"My arrest was just before the evening meal was served. At that moment, as I recall, I was sitting there looking out the window. There wasn't much to see—just other buildings. You could see walls and windows. No ground. A little sky. It was raining.

"A couple people have asked me, 'Well, when she came up to you with this medication why'd you let her do it?' Well, I don't know. I was always getting medication. I didn't realize this was any different.

"So when she came to give me this injection, I didn't think anything of it."

He refused to describe the nurse, indicating that it might interfere with the prosecution. But he volunteered: "She wasn't someone from outside."

Presumably this meant she was from the ICU.

"They [meaning the people there at the time] were the same as those who always work there—at least I didn't see anybody different.

"I think she had the syringe in her hand when she came up to the bed ... I can't recall if she said anything to me ... It didn't look funny. Nothing looked outside routine."

McCrery's note has never been made public. But the nickname on it—according to federal investigators, physicians who claim to have seen it and newspapers quoting inside sources—is "PI," or "PIA."

Goodenday had never heard the name before, she says.

"In particular, I didn't know the nurse who had been standing by his bed when the arrest occurred. [Subsequently Goodenday has said she's not even sure what the nurse looked like.] But now that he had identified her—in terms of his own protection—I felt it important that we find out who she was."

She decided to check the duty roster.

The nickname, not surprisingly, wasn't there.

Then she went to McCrery's medication chart. Nothing was charted.

McCrery, according to the record, had received no medication in the late afternoon.

"If he had been given something intravenously and it wasn't charted, that was extremely unusual," she says.

If there was a moment when Goodenday seriously began to consider the arrests possible murder attempts, this was probably it.

Certainly uneasy, she pocketed the note.

Meanwhile, upstairs, the killer (or killers), it appears, had struck again.

Upon leaving the ICU resuscitations and going up to the fifth floor, the first thing Bishop had run into was a fourth resuscitation.

"As I went back up on the wing, 5 West, I found some interns and med students working on a patient with severe chronic illness. He was in a private room. I don't remember his name or age. But he had a neurologic [organic] problem and we hadn't been able to do much for him. He survived that night but I think he died several days later."

Because this patient's arrest was approximately right after the three in the ICU, federal investigators are suspicious of it. VA doctors, however, are not. They say his poor health explains it.

The patient appears to have been Russell Fletcher, subsequently named in an indictment about the murders.

But the next arrest was more suspicious.

Leaving the unnamed patient's room, Bishop went to a four-bed area nearby. Upon entering the area, he discovered an ominously still patient. Joseph C. Brown—

the only death that day among the five afternoon arrests—was dead.

Brown, an eighty-three-year-old foundry worker from the Detroit suburb of Belleville, had acute heart and kidney trouble, and doctors didn't expect him to live long. But following a recent treatment, he'd rallied, says Bishop. And at the time he was found "we'd thought he was doing pretty well, considering.

"We hadn't expected him to die that day."

There was a "minimum sign of disturbance" surrounding Brown's death, says Bishop. The patients near him hadn't even noticed anything was wrong. There had been no chance of resuscitation. Brown was unrevivable when discovered. Bishop says he just "pulled Brown's curtain." The time of demise on Brown's death certificate is 5:50 P.M., approximately the same time that Dr. Goodenday was downstairs talking to McCrery.

Months later, federal investigators would say that a suspect in the case was seen outside what appears to have been Brown's room shortly before he was discovered.

Back downstairs, Hill, Freier and the others were finished with the antidote reversals around 6 P.M. It was probably shortly afterward that Dr. Strumpf, who had been the first physician to notice Loesch's arrest, talked to Hill briefly.

"I was told about the nerve-stimulation test," he recalls, "and that it probably confirmed that the arrests were drug-induced. I was shocked. But I had heard that they'd used neostigmine, and I wanted to find out what my intern, who was on that night, should do if another arrest occurred—should he call Dr. Hill or administer the antidote?

"It was a quick conversation. She said don't use the antidote, that they were going to talk over the situation. She said not to use it because it's not a safe drug unless you know about it and know it well. I'm sure she was concerned about someone who really didn't have the syndrome getting the antidote and being hurt by it."

Presumably standing in a hall at the time of the conversation, he adds, "Intellectually I could believe what they'd found. But emotionally I couldn't. Murder! It was almost inconceivable. But then I started reflecting back on some of the arrests I'd had and I said, 'Son of a bitch, they fall in that category.'"

The AP story about Hill indicates that she then went upstairs to her office for a few moments.

"I wanted to be alone," the story quotes her as saying.

But by approximately 6:30 P.M., it is reported, Hill was in Bishop's office, along with Bishop, Freier and, shortly, Goodenday. The office would become the "command center" (in Bishop's words) for the rest of the night.

Undoubtedly Goodenday's note, when she showed it to the others, caused a shock. Now, on top of what they'd witnessed earlier in the ICU, they had a possible suspect.

Freier says none of the others knew "PI" or "PIA" either. They called in a nursing supervisor. The supervisor told them the nickname belonged to a soft-spoken, twenty-nine-year-old nurse named Filipina Narciso. The nickname (her lawyer later speculated) was a play on Filipina.

Filipina, like several other nurses in and around the ICU, was Philippine.

Exactly what discussion followed is not known. Those in Bishop's office understandably are reluctant to get specific. Possibly there was talk of motive. Certainly there was much bafflement. But after probable suspicion of the foreign-born nurse, they must have also, upon second thought, realized that McCrery, having undergone the trauma of arrest and possibly affected by his illness or medications, might have made a mistake.

The identification must have posed a considerable dilemma.

Whatever was said, within a few minutes it appears that the foursome had decided they indeed had a probable criminal matter on their hands and that they should call in the hospital director, Arnold Mouish. As chief officer of the Ann Arbor VA, Mouish, a stocky administrator who resembles Henry Kissinger, would have to initiate the next step.

Mouish says he had been on leave in California for two weeks previous to August 15, and had only returned to work that morning. But apparently he had left the hospital for home before the arrests had begun.

Mouish lives in a house on the VA complex, but trying to reach him by phone, Freier got no answer.

Freier called an assistant administrator, and the two of them began hunting for the director.

Meanwhile, it had occurred to someone in the office, probably Hill, that they should go back down to the ICU and take urine and blood samples from the first three arrest victims.

During the earlier resuscitation of McCrery, Goodenday, acting apparently on her initial fear of contamination, had snatched McCrery's IV bag from its rack and thrust it into Bishop's hands suggesting it be analyzed.

Now they all realized they'd probably need more samples.

Hill left.

It is not certain, but it was probably during this time—when Hill went back to the ICU to take the samples—that she had the following conversation with Dr. Weber.

Weber, in addition to having performed several of the intubations, had been present during the earlier reversals and now was as concerned as the others.

"Anne had been upstairs with Freier, Bishop and Dr. Goodenday," he recalls, "and had come back to document—write on the charts—exactly what she'd done. There's a nurses' conference room just off the ICU. We were both beat. We went in and poured some coffee. I spoke first.

"I said, 'Anne, what is going on here?' She said—I can't remember her exact words—but it was something to the effect that there was a psychotic loose in the hospital who was injecting people with pancuronium or curare.

"I'm sure she used the word 'psychotic' and probably some stronger language.

"I was scared, and I think Anne was scared ... There had been no reason for the arrests and then with the nerve-stimulation tests, why we knew that there was somebody deliberately injecting the stuff.

"I said, 'I'm afraid you're right. That's what we've been thinking all along. We didn't want to believe it. I'm afraid that's what it is.'

"We sat there and finished our coffee.

Back in Bishop's office, Mouish was finally contacted, and came in around 8 to 9 P.M. By this time, all the samples were drawn and locked in a drawer in Bishop's desk. And the hospital pharmacist and chief nurse had been summoned.

Five months later, the chief nurse, Gloria J. Nunley, would recall in a newspaper story picking up her telephone that night and hearing the plea "We need you."

She must have rushed over.

Mouish, forty-nine, the former chief administrator of

the Battle Creek and Houston VA hospitals, will not discuss the Pavulon murders except in generalities. But when he came in that night, he says, "it was the first I had ever heard of the problem."

He must have been the most shocked of all.

"God, we didn't know what it was," he says of his initial briefing in Bishop's office. But his chiefs were "concerned," he adds, so "we put our heads together."

After hearing everything, Mouish was apparently impressed that something very serious had occurred. But still hoping that somehow they might have missed an explanation, the group decided they'd make one last attempt at contamination as a possible explanation.

Bishop recalls that they went to the hospital's drug storeroom and began checking the supply of IV bags to see if somehow something might have happened that they hadn't thought of.

"The IVs were in plastic bags with a parchment cover over that. We were looking to see if any seals had been broken. We were also looking at the distribution of the bags. The victims [in the ICU] didn't all have the same solutions, and we were looking to see if by some coincidence the different solutions were side by side."

But everything was intact, he says. "No seals were broken and we just didn't find anything."

There was also the remote possibility that the bags had been contaminated without the seals being broken.

"Under certain conditions," says Bishop, "some of these plastics will become permeable to certain substances. We didn't know for sure what we were dealing with. We wondered if a gaseous material could have penetrated the containers."

But again they found everything as it should have been.

Still, there was a final contamination possibility. All

the IVs were made by the same out-of-state company. Perhaps they'd been contaminated there?

They made a long-distance call, reaching one of the company's executives, presumably at home.

Mouish recalls: "I wasn't too strong on this because I felt if that were the case then we should have been experiencing the arrests during the day—you follow? I mean the IVs are dispensed continually, not just at night.

"But I wanted to give it the benefit of the doubt. So my chief and I got on the phone and we got this expert and we gave him the pattern."

Bishop recalls: "He convinced us the odds were one in ten million of a plant-caused accident. Different solutions come from different [assembly] lines. They are then stored in different warehouses hither and yon. To have a contaminated batch then come back together again in the same hospital—and on the same ward and at the same time like had happened that afternoon—was impossible."

Theirs was also the first inquiry about possible plant contamination, the executive told the hospital officials. This was further evidence that what they were suggesting was extremely improbable.

On the other hand, after a quick survey of the drugs and procedures for handling them was completed, it was determined that Pavulon was freely available in the ICU. It was kept in accessible refrigerators and unlocked drug cabinets.

There have even been confirmed reports that syringes containing Pavulon were left on ICU tables, and that partially used vials of the relaxer—with portions of the drug still in them—could be picked up in ICU garbage pails.

By 9:30 P.M., Mouish, mindful that the VA was a federal enclave, had ordered that the FBI be called.

Chapter 11

Donna Rosene Leff, brown-haired, twenty-six-year-old Ypsilanti *Press* reporter, was working late Friday, August 15. It was her turn to prepare the paper's daily obituary column, traditionally a job for beginning reporters, but on the *Press*—a small paper covering the Ypsi-Ann Arbor area—even senior staffers periodically had to take on the chore.

Donna, a Northwestern journalism graduate from Chicago, had worked for some of the country's finest papers. In the seven years previous, she had been an intern on the *Wall Street Journal*, a reporter for *Chicago Today* and a reporter and copy chief for the Chicago *Tribune*. She had come to Ypsilanti because her husband, a young Pennsylvania-born physician, wanted to train in the University of Michigan medical residency program.

Routinely telephoning funeral homes that night, she wasn't expecting anything out of the ordinary. Perhaps two thirds of the way through her calls, however, a mortuary employee suddenly said something that pricked her interest.

"They had another one [death] at the VA," she recalls him volunteering.

"You mean they've had others recently?"

"Heck yes," is an approximation of the answer. "Let me put it this way: if I got sick I'd go across town before going to the VA."

She asked several more questions. And by the time she hung up, she says, she realized the situation needed investigation. A hospital having an abnormal number of deaths was a possible story—a possible big story.

"Normally I would have called the hospital. But it was late and we were in a hurry to get out," she says. "Also, Alan [her husband] was working at the VA. He was one of the UM residents rotating there. When I got home I could check with him."

But it was nearly 3 A.M. when she finally unlocked her front door, she says, and Alan, scheduled for rounds at the VA the next morning, was asleep. Rather than wake him, she decided to wait until morning. As she got ready for bed, however, she recalled some phone calls Alan had received the night before.

"We had just gotten home. It was late. He received three quick calls from two different interns. I heard him say things like 'What? ... Who? ... He what? ... No, I'd never guess that one ... How am I supposed to know?'

"At the time I hadn't thought much about it and Alan hadn't explained because patient-doctor relations are confidential. But obviously—later I found out—they had called to tell him about some deaths and arrests. They were his interns, and they were reporting what had happened."

The calls had come on Thursday night, the fourteenth, the night Green, Ogle and Oulds had died and Drs. Zibrak and Mcleod had frantically revived Oelberg and Hall.

"I still didn't suspect murder," says Donna, "but communicable disease came to mind."

She went to sleep anxious to talk to her husband.

But Alan, a senior resident in internal medicine, was up and off the next morning before she awoke.

He recalls: "I'd heard about Friday's afternoon arrests, but I didn't suspect anything more serious than contamination. Then Saturday morning I saw Dr. Bishop in an elevator. Kind of lightly I said, 'Hey, I hear we've got a little problem here.' He got red and said, 'Shhhhhhh.' Then, when the doors closed, he told me frankly—straight out—that he thought people were being killed. I had been kind of boisterous about it until then. Then I thought, 'Oh my God, I hope nobody heard me.'"

When he got back home, Donna was waiting for him.

She recalls: "I said, 'What's going on?' And he said, 'Something weird.' I can't tell you the rest of the conversation, but suffice it to say he certainly confirmed that I should stop messing around and get to the bottom of it.

"He had a tremendous ethical problem. On the one hand he was not supposed to talk about patients or what was going on at the hospital. On the other hand, if there was murder—and it looked like there was—then wasn't there an ethical consideration there too?

"In the end," says Donna, "we concluded it would be best that I get my information from somebody else."

By the time Donna got to work that afternoon, she says, "I had made up my mind what I was going to do. There was no way in hell I was going to look the other way, both because it was too good a story and because there indeed was a compelling need to tell the story."

She now had a possible good source in mind other

than her husband. "I had never met him, but he was in a position to know."

She decided to give him a call.

"I was floored that he didn't say go to hell. In fact he kind of encouraged me. But he suggested that anything I was going to print should come from Mouish and Freier. They were in charge."

She next called Mouish.

"I put the question to him—is there anything out of the ordinary going on in the hospital? . . . Why so many deaths? . . . Why is the FBI there? [a fact she had learned in her earlier investigations]. He said, 'Oh, no, you're mistaken. Our calling the FBI is just routine. The VA is on a federal reserve and so we have to call them whenever we have anything to be investigated. It's just routine.'"

Mouish denies the accusation of a cover-up. But at least five stories from three different newspapers the following week contained statements attributed to him that the investigation was "absolutely not criminal," that it was "routine" and that the recent deaths at the hospital were "not unexpected."

He says he was misquoted.

"I was furious," says Donna. "I called my source back. He was not particularly helpful. I'd guaranteed him anonymity but he still didn't trust me fully."

At this point, Donna still didn't have enough information—or confirmation of the information she already had—to write a story. She still didn't know precisely what was going on. She called her city editor, Tom Marquardt. After hearing what she'd already found out, he too was intrigued. It was decided that the two of them would go together to the hospital. Perhaps there they could learn more.

"When we got there I was amazed at how open everything was," says Marquardt. "We walked right in the ICU and I went up to a bed. People were walking around but nobody even seemed to notice me. Then when we introduced ourselves to the nurses, there seemed to be an almost immediate sense of recognition and they said all answers would have to come from downstairs."

The two went downstairs but were met with similar refusals.

Someone then called Mouish.

Half an hour to forty-five minutes later the director arrived with Dr. Freier. Apparently Mouish had called his chief surgeon and asked him to come in with him.

The four went into Mouish's first-floor office.

"When Mouish had first come in he said he was going to tell us everything," says Donna. "But when we started questioning them they denied anything serious was going on. Their explanation was that there was a minor problem and since the staff was so busy they had to call in some help.

"I as much as called them liars. Freier played dumb. Mouish just denied everything and kept telling us what a wonderful hospital it was. It went on like that for forty-five minutes."

Marquardt recalls: "I remember I repeatedly asked Dr. Freier if he was satisfied with the way everything had been going in the ICU—that there were no problems. This was one thing I wanted to find out.

"He said yes, as far as he knew the unit was operating 'above par' ... Mr. Mouish agreed."

Mouish again denies that he wasn't frank.

"We gave her [Donna Leff] all the information we had ... We didn't know precisely what had happened ... We still don't know ... It could have been drug incompatibility, drug contamination or technique ... We didn't know."

As to the statement that he said everything was

routine, he says he told the two that it was "routine" for him to call in the FBI on an "important" case, and if they thought he meant by that that the case itself was routine, they were mistaken.

But Freier says: "We didn't really have any idea of what to discuss with the papers—how open and frank we should be. So we played cat and mouse with them.

"They would ask why had we called in the FBI. And we would say simply because they are our police force and we wanted an investigation. 'Well, why do you want an investigation?' [the reporters asked.] This went on and on.

"We didn't say much and they weren't very happy with the situation. They were primarily concerned with a big story and we were trying to hide it. But we really weren't trying to hide it as much as we had no idea what to say at that point. We knew what the impact would be ... and the matter was under investigation and we didn't want to do anything that would harm the investigation."

When they arrived back at the newspaper office, says Donna, "we had a problem. We had no official confirmation—no clear confirmation of what the story really was. We also had a problem that we were the Ypsi *Press* and not the New York *Times*, that our story had best be accurate and that we needed good attribution. Plus, there was the problem of exposing Alan and our relationship. I didn't want to damage his career."

She called her inside source one more time. But he wouldn't go on the record.

What if he was wrong? What if he himself was lying?

Donna really didn't know him.

They tried to reach the FBI but were unsuccessful.

Donna says she thought the local police might know

something, but now the reporters were afraid of something else.

"There was now a new element we had to contend with: competition. We'd been doing a lot of calling and snooping. If we called the Ann Arbor police they might very well tell the Ann Arbor *News*."

After what must have been some consternation, the *Press* decided to hold the story over the weekend.

"In retrospect it seems a preposterous decision," says Donna, "but at the time, we felt we could probably sit on it."

When Donna finally arrived home Saturday night, August 16, there was a party going on. Some of Alan's doctor friends were there.

"We got to shooting the breeze. I told them what I knew. They confirmed it and even gave me some numbers, forty-one arrests and seven deaths. [The figures, she would later write, were for the three-week period beginning July 28.] I eventually got enough details that I knew I could nail it on Monday morning no matter what.

"At that point I was a nervous wreck. I just knew one of the other papers would have it in the morning. Here we were discussing it at a party!"

But Sunday came and there wasn't a mention. Monday morning it was the same thing.

Apparently nobody else had gotten wind of the investigation.

The *Press* is an afternoon daily. Donna was at her desk early Monday morning. At approximately 8:50 A.M., according to an official government memorandum, she called VA headquarters in Washington.

The memo reads: "Ms. Donna Leff, reporter for the Ypsilanti *Press*, telephoned to inquire about an alleged increase in respiratory arrests at the [Ann Arbor VA]. [Even Washington, it appears, didn't know yet.] She advised that her information was that ... forty-one patients [had suffered respiratory arrests and] seven of the forty-one ... expired as a result ... According to Ms. Leff all the patients ... were receiving IVs ... [and] the FBI had been called into the case to investigate if the IV solutions had been altered by person—persons—unknown.

Ms. Leff advised that she met with ... Arnold Mouish ... Mr. Mouish acknowledged that the FBI had been called in ... admitted 'some concern,' but denied being alarmed ... [She] claims to have spoken with a member of the regular medical staff at the [hospital, her source, who] is alleged to have ... found the whole situation unusual ... She ... has a number of questions which she ... would like to have answered before [writing] her story."

She would call back in an hour, the memo ends.

Meanwhile, at the hospital, med chief Bishop, concerned that no one had told the rank-and-file doctors what was happening, had called a special meeting Monday morning of the institution's house staff: interns, residents and fellows.

"I don't remember specifically what I said," Bishop recalls. "I just asked them to gather and told them what I knew."

Most of the doctors were stunned.

"I give him a lot of credit," says Dr. Eric Hodeen, a fellowship holder in rheumatoid diseases and president of the House Officers Association, the organization of all University of Michigan house staff, including those at the VA. "There is a tendency many times on the part of the administration and chiefs of services to ignore the house staff. But Dr. Bishop was fairly open. He told us what had been going on."

Alan Leff, one of the physicians attending the meeting, recalls: "There was a lot of disbelief and denial. They couldn't believe what they were hearing."

Being already familiar with the situation, Leff was one of the first to react.

"I said, 'Listen, I don't know how the rest of you feel, but I'm being told by the head of medicine here that he thinks our patients are being murdered and I'm unwilling to bring any patients into the hospital.'"

He proposed that they demand that the administration stop all admissions.

"The worst we can do by this is look foolish. The best is prevent a murder ... How can we sweep this under the rug?"

It was an almost unheard-of proposal. If they stopped all admissions, there was a chance critically ill people might die.

The issue was discussed. Finally, a vote was called. The result was that the majority agreed with Leff—except in extreme emergencies.

"Not a rule-out appendicitis [a widely-used term for undiagnosed abdominal pain]" recalls Leff. "It would have to be someone with a ruptured appendix—only cases where death was imminent if [they were] not admitted and treated."

In addition, the group voted to demand that the hospital inform all present patients of the investigation and provide emergency cases with a written statement of the chances they might be taking by entering.

The hospital had already instituted certain safeguards. Friday night, for instance, Mouish had ordered all drugs locked up and extra personnel, including more security guards, into the ICU and the hospital's halls. But this would be a much larger step.

A committee of three senior residents, including Leff and Hodeen, was appointed by the house staff to present the demands to the administration. Hodeen, because he was president of the larger association, was designated spokesman. Sometime that morning, the committee, accompanied by Bishop, went to Mouish's office.

What happened next is unclear.

Hodeen and Leff say that at first Mouish and aides were reluctant to agree to the recommendations.

"They said they'd already taken some precautionary steps," recalls Hodeen, "but they didn't seem ready to take the step of saying emergencies only ... I think they thought it was too drastic.

"To be very candid, I don't think they would have agreed unless we'd applied some subtle pressure; we told them we'd tell the press what we'd voted unless they agreed."

Mouish says he doesn't remember any reluctance.

"You'll find all kinds of experts after the fact," he says. "We were perplexed and we discussed some possibilities that would make things more livable, one of which was to get some kind of communication out to the patients and another which was to consider limiting admissions."

Bishop doesn't remember a "confrontation." But an administrative aide, Gary Calhoun, says Hodeen and Leff are essentially correct.

"You've got to understand what a decision that is," he explains.

Whatever the case, shortly thereafter the hospital began to limit admissions on a large scale. By Tuesday, for instance, according to newspaper figures (and again it must be stressed that the hospital will not provide official records to non-government researchers), the patient population dropped to 260 from Monday's 285.

In her newspaper office, Donna Leff was aware of the house staff meeting. Another *Ypsi* reporter, John Barton, had also finally received FBI confirmation of a probe at the hospital of at least one "unexplained" death.

The two facts were all she needed to complete her story.

At 10:36 A.M., according to the official memo at VA headquarters, she called Washington back, asking if they had any information for her. The author of the memo advised her to contact "information service," the VA's public relations arm.

She disregarded the ploy.

Probably around 11 A.M. she turned to her typewriter and began writing the story which would eventually win her several awards and her newspaper much prestige.

Copyrighted by the Ypsi *Press,* it began:

"The Federal Bureau of Investigation is investigating at least one unexplained death and reviewing forty-one other cases involving respiratory arrests at the Veterans Administration Hospital in Ann Arbor.

"Arnold E. Mouish, administrator of the hospital, confirmed today that the VA facility is limiting admissions to emergencies.

"A dramatic upsurge in respiratory arrest cases has caused alarm among hospital staff members and new admissions were stopped today until the causes of the problem can be determined."

She was hedging on calling the arrests criminal, but the shocking possibilities glared through:

"Whether the deaths were accidental, natural or otherwise has not been determined . . . Sources say all intravenous tubes and fluids used to treat stricken patients have been collected and are being analyzed for 'foreign substances' . . . Another source said he disagreed with statements by the hospital administration that the investigation was 'routine.' "

The story was to cause pandemonium.

Chapter 12

At first the wire services were skeptical of the Ypsi story. The *Press* was a small paper. The facts might be incorrect.

They decided to put the story on the state wire, but not the national wire.

Papers, television and radio stations outside Michigan wouldn't get it.

But state circulation was enough.

Sometime Monday, editors of the Detroit *Free Press*, one of the best newspapers in the respected Knight chain, received the story. Skeptical too, they nevertheless asked a reporter to check it out.

The reporter, Maryanne Conheim, called Mouish. The administrator, her subsequent story says, denied all "rumors" of foul play.

"They've all been extremely ill," she quoted him as saying about the recent deaths. "They've all been elderly. These deaths were not unexpected."

But the FBI, Conheim wrote, said, "We are not an agency that does things for the hell of it. We would not be involved unless circumstances indicated it was warranted."

It was enough to make the *Free Press* suspicious, and what the *Free Press* wrote *would* be carried across the nation.

But like the Ypsi *Press,* the *Free Press,* too, didn't yet have enough information to call the deaths murder. So Conheim wrote a story reacting to the Ypsi intimations.

Conheim's article, which appeared Tuesday morning, August 19, began: "The FBI confirmed Monday that it is probing forty-one cases of respiratory failure—including seven deaths—within the last three weeks at the Veterans Administration Hospital in Ann Arbor..."

In addition, the story contained the Ypsi paper's quote of a "doctor on the hospital staff" saying, even though Mouish maintained the investigation was routine, "I have never been interviewed by the FBI before."

Tuesday afternoon the Ypsi *Press*'s second story on the hospital hit the streets. Donna Leff and a small company of reporters had by then learned that a muscle relaxer was the suspect drug in the deaths and arrests, and that an investigatory VA team from Washington was arriving that day.

The Detroit *News,* the area's other large daily, ran its first story on the hospital deaths Tuesday afternoon. It too reported the imminent arrival of the VA headquarters team, and, for the first time in any newspaper, quoted Mouish as saying the investigation was something other than normal.

"The situation is serious enough to look at and evaluate," *News* reporter Peter Lochbiler wrote that the administrator had told him, "although it is not completely outside our previous experience."

Meanwhile, at the *Free Press,* editors still weren't satisfied. They decided to send two of their best young reporters to Ann Arbor—forty-five minutes' drive from Detroit—to see what a team could dig up.

Kirk Cheyfitz, twenty-eight, had come to the paper from his native Washington, D.C., area. Jim Schutze, thirty, had grown up in Ann Arbor and graduated from the University of Michigan.

Both reporters were smart and aggressive.

"We were excited about the story," recalls blond-bearded Schutze. "We sensed it was big. We had separate cars with radios. I remember talking and planning about what we were going to do as we rode down the freeway."

When they reached the Ann Arbor turnoffs, Cheyfitz went directly to the VA. Schutze went into town to the University of Michigan hospital.

"I had a friend there," he recalls. "I knew he wouldn't be officially involved and so maybe he could tell me something."

The friend didn't know much, says Schutze, but he volunteered that he knew someone who did—a department head who was testing something for the investigation from the VA.

Sometime late Friday, August 15, one of the Ann Arbor VA's pharmacy officials had hand-carried some of the samples taken from the patients stricken that afternoon to the University of Michigan hospital lab. It was these samples that the department head was testing.

Schutze went up to see him.

"In talking with the guy, he said, 'You know of course that we think we've found Pavulon.' I said, 'Oh yes, I know about that.' Of course I didn't know anything. I didn't even know what Pavulon was. But I went on like I did, and eventually he explained it all to me.

"When we were through, I asked him three times,

'Now if it's Pavulon, could it possibly be an accident?' Each time he said no. So I said, 'Okay, then you're telling me that somebody over there is killing people.' And he said, 'Well, if that's what you want to call it. It's really a spooky scene.' "

Schutze was already suspecting something drastic. Now he had it from a sterling source. Not only was the man a respected UM researcher, but he didn't know Schutze was coming and, being unattached to the VA, he was neutral in the controversy.

Schutze went to his car and sped to the VA.

Cheyfitz was on the front steps when he pulled up.

Cheyfitz, too, had heard about some tests—a "gas chromatograph," a chemical analysis. It indicated that some of the arrests might have been caused by a muscle relaxer.

Apparently, the two decided, it was the same information Schutze had just learned.

"Suddenly we realized we had a helluva story," says Schutze.

They devised a loose plan. Schutze went in to try and gather more information from the interns and residents. Cheyfitz went directly to Mouish's first-floor office.

By this time, the Washington VA team had arrived. Heading it was Dr. Laurance V. Foye, Jr., a stocky, bespectacled administrator. Foye was in Mouish's office.

"Mouish and I started talking," says Cheyfitz. "I told him I knew about the tests and he said that was a lie, that I was going to write something based on rumor and untruth.

"We got into a screaming match. In the middle he said, 'All right, I'm going to get Dr. Bishop down here and he's going to tell you it's a lie.'

"I said fine."

When Cheyfitz had arrived at the hospital earlier, the resident who told him about the tests had indicated that it was Bishop who had seen the gas chromatograph. During the argument, Cheyfitz had interjected Bishop's name, and that apparently was why Mouish was calling for him.

"Mouish called me in there," recalls Bishop. "Dr. Foye from the central office was there, and he [Mouish] wanted me to tell Cheyfitz that there was nothing in the fluid [McCrery's IV fluid, which was the subject of the gas chromatograph].

"I just wouldn't do it . . . I'd seen the graph. I'd seen the little blip that indicated an impurity . . ."

The testers had tentatively labeled the impurity succinylcholine, a muscle relaxer very similar to Pavulon, says Bishop. But either succinylcholine or Pavulon (pancuronium) could have caused the blip, he says, "and as far as I was concerned it was wrong to say there was nothing there."

It was a "traumatic experience," Bishop recalls of his predicament between the two sides. "I couldn't say this was off the record or anything like that. Cheyfitz was asking me cold blank, 'What is it?'"

He says he drew a picture of the graph showing where the impurity showed up.

"Foye looked at Mouish," he says, "and said, 'My goodness, Arnold, is this really true? Have we really got this?' And I said, 'Why, yes, [the pharmacist] has the graph.'"

Mouish says: "At the time we had that discussion with Cheyfitz we had absolutely no official record from the pharmacology lab . . . There were some informal grapevine reports but, hell, you know you can't operate on that . . . [The graph] was extremely inconclusive and could not be used in any way, shape or form."

Foye says: "I think Mouish was trying to hold down

the hysteria level. Kirk [Cheyfitz] is very aggressive and was trying to push him into saying something he was not sure of."

Mouish was right. The tests *were* inconclusive. But Cheyfitz had heard what he wanted. Bishop wasn't denying that there was a muscle relaxer involved. In fact, he was admitting it.

The administration was rapidly losing its credibility.

Elsewhere in the hospital, Schutze was trying to interview patients. When Cheyfitz emerged from Mouish's office he told Schutze what had just happened and the two went looking for Hodeen, the House Officers Association president who, the day before, had also had a disagreement with Mouish.

"I didn't really know exactly what we'd have to say," recalls Schutze. "I thought maybe we'd have to give him a rough time. But he was very straight. He said, 'Glad to have you here.' His only thing was that he wanted these patients to know what was going on. He kept saying, 'We don't want the patients to be endangered.'"

As far as he knew, the reporters say Hodeen told them, "these patients were not dying of natural causes," and the administration was just being a "scared bureaucracy"—afraid of bad publicity—in saying that they were.

It was another confirmation.

But they still wanted more.

Since it was approaching their deadline, 4:30 P.M., it was decided that Schutze would go back to the office and begin writing, and Cheyfitz would remain to see what else he could get.

Finding another member of the Washington team— one of lesser title than Foye—Cheyfitz maneuvered him into a corner.

"I told him what we knew: the tests, the probable

presence of a muscle relaxer, the clinical impressions that the doctors were telling us about.

"I said, 'You know the FBI is convinced it's murder and I know you're convinced it's murder. Now what is it?'

"He said, off the record, 'It's murder.'"

It was the best confirmation yet.

Cheyfitz says he phoned it in to Schutze and then "drove like hell for the paper."

When he arrived, Schutze had just finished the story and turned it in.

The lead he had carefully typed said: "ANN ARBOR—All non-emergency surgery was halted at the Veterans Hospital here Tuesday as investigators said there was a possibility that someone in the hospital may be using paralyzing drugs in an attempt to murder patients."

It was the first time the word "murder" had been used in a newspaper story about the arrests and deaths, and some *Free Press* executives were skeptical.

"It was a heavy scene," Schutze recalls. "We were convinced it was murder, but our editors were looking at it and saying, 'Yeah, that's a great story, but it ain't true.' No one had said 'murder' for the record and we had a big fight with them."

Finally, however, the editors relented.

Schutze recalls: "Jennie Buckner, the assistant city editor—the same one who sent us over there in the first place because she knew it was too good a story to kiss off on the phone—came over and said, 'Okay, I hope you guys are right, because the news desk wants to put it on page one.'

"We said, 'We know we are.'"

The story also contained one of the first informed body counts.

Spotlighting statistics which, according to Cheyfitz, had been picked up mostly "looking over people's shoulders, copying down lists and demanding things under the Freedom of Information Act, which the [hospital] administration didn't seem to understand," the story included: "The hospital has had 34 [newspaper accounts, using different sources, have right up to the present printed varying figures] cases of respiratory arrest—total loss of breathing—involving 23 patients in the last three weeks, according to Dr. Lawrence [sic] Foye, Jr., head of a team of medical investigators flown in Tuesday . . . Eight of the patients have died."

When the story appeared Wednesday morning under the headline KILLER AT LARGE IN VETERANS HOSPITAL? virtually every major news-gathering agency in the nation took note. The *Free Press* is not a small paper.

Within hours, television crews, special correspondents and radio broadcasters were swarming through the hospital's halls deluging everyone they could with questions.

"The place was swarming with CBS and NBC and, gosh, men running around all over the place," recalls one patient's wife. "And boy, they [the hospital] had guards all over, and the reporters were trying to get through and the guards were pushing them back. It was a madhouse."

It was like a "circus," says Schutze. "Everyone was running around trying to get information. Flashbulbs were popping. People were pushing. TV cameras would hit you in the back. There were some funny scenes too.

"The administration wouldn't let you interview patients in the hospital. So whenever one of them would go outside for sun or anything he'd get chased around. As soon as one of them would start talking, other reporters would come running over.

"I remember one guy started talking freely and everyone rushed over. He was saying something about the CIA and we were all listening intently. But after about ten sentences we realized he was nuts. He was a psycho patient."

Cheyfitz, an aspiring film maker, remembers it looked like a "movie set—national networks flying in crews from Chicago and New York—that sort of thing." He says he casually mentioned this to a Detroit television newsman standing near him and the newsman, mistaking him for a hospital official complaining about the press presence, became hostile, demanding to know what he thought was wrong.

But for some of the patients it was a deadly serious and, in some cases, traumatic experience.

The hospital, for instance, had still not told patients exactly what was going on.

A U.S. Government memorandum, addressed to "all patients," and eventually passed out, said:

"You have probably heard rumors about the occurrence of ill patients suddenly developing breathing difficulty in the past two and a half weeks. We are continuing a complete investigation of the circumstances surrounding these incidents and we would appreciate any help that you can give the investigators. There have been no episodes of this nature in the last four days. There has been an increase in staffing and supervision with respect to the control of certain medications and we feel that there should be no further occurrence of this problem.

"Rest assured that we will continue in every way to deliver the best possible medical care to our patients."

But the memo hardly could be called candid.

Most patients learned about the darker side of the story—the probability that there was a maniac loose in the hospital—through the morning *Free Press* article or from one of the newsmen that rushed to the VA after its appearance.

"I heard about it on the radio," recalls Mrs. Lutz, whose husband suffered several of the mysterious arrests in late July. "It nearly flipped me."

She says she rushed to the hospital, was confronted with newspaper reporters on the steps and had to push her way through a mob inside to get upstairs to where her husband was.

"When I got there they had given out a sheet of paper to all the patients that said something had happened and that everybody would probably be interviewed. We didn't even keep it."

Presumably this was the government memorandum.

Mrs. Lutz complains—and it is a complaint voiced by many of the families involved—that one of the confusing things about those days was that the hospital never told her that her husband was one of the patients suspected of having suffered a Pavulon attack.

"They never told us anything."

In fact, as late as early summer 1976—eleven months after the attacks—the families of patients suspected of suffering Pavulon attacks still had not been notified.

And a good number of those patients are dead.

Mouish says: "We did not have the time to write or telephone or contact all next of kin. And the relatives getting upset is one of the disadvantages of premature reporting by newspapers.

"Even today we still don't know who was a victim. The newspapers have talked in terms of ten deaths, twelve deaths, possibly thirty. So far as we know, we think we have had one death and even that is not conclusive.

"So how can we notify when we don't know?"

Conservative estimates at the time of Mouish's statement (1976) were placing the death toll at a probable six.

In an editorial August 30, 1975, the Ypsi *Press* said it was "disgusted and mortified by the Veterans Administration's lack of sensitivity for the families of recently deceased patients.

"We can understand, of course, the hospital's reluctance to establish liability in these bizarre cases. However, there has to be a middle position between accepting blame for some of the unexplained deaths and having the human decency to supply comfort to very concerned families."

But with the swarms of newsmen and newswomen all over the hospital that Wednesday morning, the hospital eventually had to do something of substance. So it called a press conference.

One can imagine the hushed silence as VA officials made their way to a hastily constructed podium. Microphones with station identifications bristled before them. The mob of reporters—if not the occasion itself—had probably heated up the atmosphere. A newspaper picture shows Dr. Foye wiping sweat from his brow with a handkerchief.

Foye, according to published reports, was possibly coy. But he didn't deny what almost everyone now knew.

"One of the many possibilities is that it was an intentional act," one story quotes him as admitting, "but, so far, we have been unable to develop supporting evidence that this was an intentional act." The arrests and deaths were "unexpected," the story quotes him, but the tests on fluids from patients involved "are so far inconclusive."

After the conference, he told the *Free Press,* and presumably other papers as well, that chances of the arrests and deaths being accidental had been "virtually ruled out."

The conference and the remarks afterward were the

first large-scale official public recognition of a serious problem at the VA. That afternoon, the Ann Arbor *News,* larger than the Ypsilanti *Press,* but so far hesitant about the VA problem, splashed its first big VA murder story across the entire top of page one.

POISONINGS SUSPECTED IN 7 DEATHS, said the main headline. "Deliberate Act Possible," read the smaller kicker above.

A second story occupying most of the lower right of the front page was headlined SO MANY RUMORS, and praised the VA while intimating that the hospital had been wrongly maligned by speculation not based on acknowledged fact.

A column by Ypsilanti *Press* editor Tim McGuire two days later would say the AA *News* was "soft-pedaling the case." But few of the newsmen and newswomen at the press conference knew or cared about what was to become a heated and consequential competition between the local area newspapers. Most were from out of town—from large metropolitan news-gathering organizations where stories of the bizarre and chilling were prized items for their daily reports.

That evening, as viewers around the nation watched the "CBS Evening News," they heard anchorman Roger Mudd say, "A strange story is unfolding at a federal hospital in Michigan. It's a story of a mysterious death, and, according to some, possible homicide. Sharon Lovejoy reports."

Lovejoy: "The Veterans Administration Hospital in Ann Arbor, Michigan: on the surface, calm and peaceful, a haven for the sick.

"But there is fear on the loose here.

"In the space of just three weeks, twenty-three patients here have suffered respiratory failure. Eight died before they could be revived.

"The staff, at a loss to explain what has caused the abnormal number of respiratory arrests, brought in the FBI and a VA medical team. Their findings: early tests show a trace of muscle relaxant in the intravenous solution given one victim—medicine which is used to cause temporary paralysis during operations.

"Since those drugs have been put under lock and key, the incidents have stopped. But still the questions remain."

Suddenly, Foye was being interviewed on the screen.

"So far all our leads on any question of misuse of these drugs have been negative," he said. "In other words, have drugs disappeared? We are unable to document that. Has too much drug been used? We are unable to document that. Have drugs been kept where they should not be? . . . We have no evidence of that."

Lovejoy: "Worried, Mrs. Audrey Krill refused to let her husband, John, be admitted for the fitting of an artificial limb."

Mrs. Krill: "And I told him, no way in hell . . . and they said why not? And I said, right now . . . he does not need any respiratory problems. And I said with the cases you got up here, and he just does not need any more hospitalization or anything else going wrong. He's had enough."

Lovejoy: "The search for answers goes on . . ."

Rebecca Bell handled the story for NBC. "A team of FBI agents and medical specialists are interviewing members of the hospital staff and going over records today to try to determine if bizarre medical coincidence, accident, or a psychopath is killing patients at this small VA hospital," she began.

"There is no panic at the hospital, but a number of patients have, at their own request, been transferred elsewhere. The unusual number of respiratory arrest cases . . . has caused investigators to raise the possibility that someone might be administering the paralyzing drug to patients."

She, too, interviewed Foye.

Following the press conference, the hospital administration stopped talking to all but the most persistent reporters, and then only reluctantly.

Desks with guards were set up in front of the first-floor administration offices and only badge-wearing personnel were admitted freely. All inquiries were referred to designated administrative aides. Top officials withdrew to the hospital's impenetrable innards, marked "Off Limits" to outside personnel.

There was an investigation going on, and no one could be told anything, was the reply.

But the nation was now alerted. The press, for varied reasons, had probably forced disclosure of a danger that might otherwise have remained a secret a long time. And now, not only a few reporters but millions of people everywhere wanted to know who the Ann Arbor killer (or killers) was.

Chapter 13

When Special Agent Gene Ward arrived at the VA hospital that Friday evening following the August 15 afternoon respiratory arrests, he must have had many questions. Facing him was the real possibility of mass murder, so medically complex and technical that for over a month it had eluded the detection of even the hospital's top physicians.

It also, presumably, was unlike anything he'd ever investigated before.

After listening to everything those who had summoned him had to say, he made a call.

"It was such a bizarre situation," recalls Richard Delonis, thirty-four-year-old head of criminal prosecutions for the U. S. Attorney's Office, Detroit, who answered at the other end.

Ward wanted to know whether Delonis agreed a crime had been committed. Delonis, after due consideration, said he did, and that the thought of someone doing such a thing horrified him.

Delonis, Ward and a company of some twenty FBI agents were to become the fact-gatherers and decision-makers for the investigation just beginning. Few federal investigators will speak much about the case. But judging from what followed, the two men decided on an immediate probe to begin that very night.

"We knew we had an immense task," says Delonis, "and we didn't want to miss anything."

One of the first things Ward did after talking to Delonis, say those present, was to see McCrery in the ICU.

It wasn't that Ward was so impressed with McCrery's note, says Freier. In fact, it appeared to the chief surgeon that Ward would much rather have had an IV tube with fingerprints on it handed to him, or a traceable murder weapon—hard evidence indisputably putting the killer at the scene.

The note really was not that solid. A defense lawyer conceivably could present it as the mistaken scratchings of a confused patient—possibly even hearsay.

But it was all they initially had.

Gary Calhoun, the hospital administrative assistant, remembers going to the ICU with Ward:

"McCrery was still intubated, and we asked him pretty much the same questions [that Goodenday had]. And he said, yeah, yes, that was true."

"You asked him? But with the intubation tube he couldn't speak."

"No, but he could still move his head and write notes."

"Did he write 'P.I.'s' name again?"

"I don't think we asked him to write it down again. He just shook his head yes to questions."

At least one more time that night, indicates Calhoun, the two visited McCrery. The next thing most of those present recall is that Ward set up a room in a lower-floor office and began interrogating ICU personnel.

It must have been obvious that if a crime had been

committed that day it was a good bet that someone working in the ICU at that time—which meant all of them—probably had done it, or at least had witnessed something pertinent.

Ward even had evidence to that effect.

If he could piece things together that night, he'd probably be able to crack the case by morning.

It was probably at this initial interrogation that Ward first confronted "P.I."—the ICU nurse Filipina Narciso—with the damaging note naming her.

Narciso, although approachable on other subjects, has been told by her lawyer, Tom O'Brien, a young Ann Arbor attorney, not to discuss the case with anyone. Several months after August 15, however, O'Brien would readily concede that his client *was* in McCrery's "vicinity" when he had his respiratory arrest. But being one of the ICU nurses, he explains, she was *supposed* to be near him.

"We understand that what happened was that during one of the other codes ... McCrery's light went on—the light that patients can self-actuate when they want someone to come. And that P.I. was on her way to get something and stopped by and he knew about the other codes in progress and [said] he was jittery about them ... And he complained his extension tubing was too short—his IV hurt him and he wanted someone to stay with him.

"The way I understand it was that it was explained to him that P.I. couldn't stay because there was another code in progress. But she switched the ... IV tubing for him—put an extension on it—and tried to make him comfortable and then went back to the code and informed his nurse, Leonie Perez [another Filipino], about the situation. And then I understand that she [Perez] went back in five minutes or so to check in on him. He was okay. She went back to the code in progress. And then I understand that sometime after that the Code 7 flashed on McCrery."

So if Narciso was questioned that night, then the above—or something like it—is probably what she related.

She denied everything.

Also, if Ward questioned her at that time, and if he did indeed have strong suspicions about her, he probably was struck by her disarming manner.

She has a soft voice and shy demeanor—almost apologetic when she talks.

She frequently appears to be smiling.

As she sat before him, as she doubtless did, it must have been difficult to picture her cold-bloodedly injecting poison into McCrery's IV.

But then again, he could have decided, a killer of this sort has got to be insane—perhaps schizophrenic. He or she easily could be hiding another face.

Narciso, for her part—if, again, she had gone before Ward, and if she was telling the truth—must have been shaken, possibly very scared.

She was an alien in a foreign country—unmarried, alone except for nursing friends, a small family group she lived with and several close neighbors.

Her parents were thousands of miles away in the Philippines.

Suddenly she was being accused of a ghastly crime: multiple attacks on helpless patients. She cared for her patients, she might have protested. How could he think such a thing of her.

It is not known how long Ward kept the ICU personnel that night. Some say practically until dawn. But that never has been verified. But even before he had started the interviews, the hospital had begun an intensive examination of its records to begin providing the FBI with accurate information.

The bureau was going to need facts—the who, what, where and why of all the respiratory arrests—not speculation, Ward probably told Mouish. Nurses then began poring over charts and folders. Eventually, this task was given over to the VA team from Washington, and, ultimately, to a committee of outside doctors, who, at two marathon sittings lasting several days the next week, debated out the following initial data:

There had been approximately fifty arrests between July 1 and August 15. Normally, the hospital could have expected about fourteen in the same period. This meant that about 35 of the fifty were above average— thirty-five possible attacks in the seven-week period.

But few of the physicians, if any, agreed with such a high estimate. It would be unreasonable, they felt, to assume that all the "above average" arrests were attacks. Rather, they drew up a list of arrests which they considered "very suspicious," "moderately suspicious," "suspicious" and "not suspicious."

At the top of the list, in the "very suspicious" category, were some fifteen arrests (give or take a few, depending on whose list it was) which the doctors felt, try as they might, could not be explained away.

The patient's illness did not signal an arrest. His medical history didn't forecast it. Nor did any of the facts surrounding the seizure, such as the medicine he was on or treatment he was receiving.

The arrests, simply, were mysteries.

If a poisoner had been operating in the hospital, the probability was that these, above all others, had been the result of his or her work.

The committee's deliberations were conducted behind closed doors. But according to some who were there—numerous VA doctors testified before the panel and otherwise aided in the sifting—the "top fifteen" included arrests suffered by Blaine, Loesch, McCrery,

Oulds, Green, Oelberg, Gasmire, Lutz, Neely and Herman, the bulk of those who had raised suspicions before August 15.

Several of the fifteen were dead. Several others would die in the next few weeks.

Undoubtedly, the killer or killers had attacked more. Perhaps there had been as many as thirty attacks and fifteen murders. And indeed the official attack and death toll would grow. But fifteen, including one or two deaths (again, depending on whose list was being consulted), was all the committee at that time could be reasonably sure of.

After the sessions, those were the initial approximate figures it handed the FBI.

As the medical chiefs were familiar with most of the arrests soon to be placed on the official top fifteen, Agent Ward probably learned about the majority of "very suspicious" arrests that very first night.

In addition, he doubtless came to another conclusion: The killer appeared to be someone with medical know-how—a doctor, a technician or a nurse. How else could a poisoner have operated so unnoticeably? Also, injection of a muscle relaxer took special medical knowledge.

First indications were that the killer had shot it into the IV tubing and not the skin.

This in itself was the mark of a professional. It was clean—and cunning. The victim hardly knew what was happening, and, depending on circumstances, it afforded the assailant time to get away. If the drug was injected up high in the tubing, for instance, it took time for it to descend.

Most of the arrests had occurred in the ICU, and at night. This pointed squarely to the night ICU staff.

Sometime early that first weekend, Ward returned to McCrery's bedside.

Under the pretense of having them show him how

McCrery's IV worked, the agent had ICU nurses go before the arrest victim so he could get a close look at them.

"They ran about four or five nurses—I can't remember exactly how many—past my bed," the Ypsilanti *Press* later quoted McCrery as saying. "They told me to look at all of them carefully and wait before picking her out.

"Now that I think about it, that made good sense ... because ... if she could tell that I knew, she might come back and try to get me again."

Who McCrery picked out is not positively known. McCrery himself is either confused about it or won't say. (The reason why will become clear later.)

But the *Press* says it was Narciso. And Gary Calhoun, who claims to have been the only other person with Ward at the time, appears to confirm that.

Declining actually to name the nurse, Calhoun nevertheless volunteers that "four times" in the four days following McCrery's attack, including the two times already mentioned, he went into McCrery's room to check on the arrest victim's testimony. And each time, he says, McCrery confirmed "the same person it has been said he identified from the start."

Also that weekend, McCrery, it seems certain, contributed at least one more incriminating note.

Dr. Joe Zibrak, the intern who helped fight the August 14 arrests and deaths, says that Saturday morning he visited McCrery, and, in response to a question, McCrery wrote that a "nurse" had attacked him. There was also other writing on the "second note," says Zibrak (the first had already been confiscated by Ward), including something about "a person of Mexican descent."

McCrery himself appears to remember the second note:

He says that later in the investigation, the FBI showed him "a sheet of paper" with lots of "questions and answers" on it—"sometimes just answers." Things were written all over it, he says, in different kinds of handwriting. "It even had something referring to a picture of a twenty-seven-pound king salmon I'd caught on the lake. I had a snapshot of it with me in the hospital and they must have asked me about it."

If—as they had told him—he had written the reference to a person of "Mexican descent" in response to a question about who had attacked him (and he guesses he did), then he made a mistake, he says.

What he meant by that, he says, was an "Oriental."

But the Oriental wasn't necessarily Narciso.

There was more than one Pacific islander in the ICU. Leonora (also called Leonie) Perez, already mentioned as McCrery's nurse in connection with Narciso's possible August 15 statement to Ward, was also Filipino and had Oriental features.

To Westerners, the two looked similar.

And there were other Oriental nurses in the unit, and elsewhere in the hospital.

Could McCrery have mixed two of them up? Perez, too, had been around McCrery at the time of the arrest, according to Narciso's lawyer.

It was a possibility.

But that first weekend of the investigation, the evidence appears to have been pointing solely at Narciso. And it doesn't appear that Ward had any other thoughts.

It's probable that he was already setting in motion the FBI machinery to determine exactly who this quiet Filipino, steadfastly maintaining her innocence, was; and whether there was anything in her past or present life suggestive of such a monstrous crime.

Chapter 14

Approximately 5'4" tall and 130 pounds, Filipina Bobadilla Narciso, her black hair cut short around her ears, was probably easy to trace. Her life, meaningful as it was for her, was, from an official records standpoint, relatively uneventful.

Although most government files about her are secret, press investigations, talks with her and interviews with her lawyer, friends and acquaintances produced the following portrait:

She was born May 17, 1946. That made her twenty-nine years, two months and twenty-nine days old on the day the investigation started. Her home was near Manila, the Philippine capital. Michigan must have been a great change for her. The Philippines are, for the most part, jungly, hot and steamy. Michigan is a state with large woodlands and long, cold winters.

World War II had only been over a matter of months when she was born. Her family was large— nine children, five girls and four boys. Her father is a retired building contractor. Both parents, probably in their sixties, are still living.

She writes them frequently, sometimes sending money.

Probably she'd had contact with American servicemen while growing up. The Philippines are still key islands in the U.S. defense system, and there were many military bases there right after World War II.

Could something have happened there to have provided a motive for the mass murders? A cruelty to herself or her family? A disgrace of some kind?

Could she have been attacking American servicemen for revenge?

It's probable that the FBI checked on this possibility. But nothing has surfaced so far to give any indication that they found anything.

One agent says: "There was some speculation about the Philippines and the war, but it didn't pan out."

It is possible, however, that the slightly built girl's plans to become a nurse in America materialized, at least partly, as a result of exposure to Americans. The Philippines have been under American control most of the time since 1898, when they were won in the Spanish-American War. A system of American hospitals had been in operation there long before World War II, and becoming a nurse through some of their training programs was—and still is, according to medical authorities—a good way to get to the United States, which itself appears to have been a desirable goal among Filipinos.

Besides, there was a market for Filipino nurses in America, says Helen Dunn, administrative secretary of the Michigan State Board of Nursing, where Narciso was registered and certain public information about her is available.

Recruiters received $1,000 "a head," and "imported them in groups."

But there is no information indicating Narciso was recruited that way.

She is a graduate of the Philippine Women's University College of Nursing in Manila, according to her records. She received the equivalent of a bachelor's degree November 8, 1969, and then studied and trained several more years, possibly for a second degree.

The Detroit *Free Press* says that Dr. Rosario Diamte, dean of the college, remembers teaching a course to Narciso. "Dr. Diamte said Miss Narciso was so average that it was difficult to remember much about her," Kirk Cheyfitz wrote.

She was licensed in the Philippines following her graduation, and then, after an approximate year and a half interval, arrived in the United States May 27, 1971, ten days following her twenty-fifth birthday.

Her point of entry to America, according to her lawyer, was Alaska. It was there, probably, that immigration officials gave her the status of "permanent resident," meaning that she told them she was planning to stay.

An immigrant first coming to America must wait five years before being given citizenship status. As a resident, she is supposed to be afforded all privileges of a citizen except voting.

But in plain language, until such citizenship is granted, she is an alien. And some would later charge that because she wasn't a full-fledged American her civil rights were forgotten when the investigation turned on her.

In the meantime, she retains her Filipino citizenship.

Once in the United States, Narciso went south to the University of Alabama in Birmingham, where she took a job at the university hospital. It was while in Birmingham, says the *Free Press*, that she acquired the nickname "P.I." which eventually was to be a factor in her incrimination. Possibly the name stood for Philippine Islands or was a diminutive of her first name. At any rate, the nickname appears to have been bestowed amicably.

Narciso spent approximately two years in Alabama. On September 29, 1972, she was granted, on the basis of testing, a higher license than she previously held—that of registered nurse. Her records say she passed her English proficiency test the first time. The conversational part of the exam is the toughest part for aliens, say nursing officials.

She moved to Ann Arbor in November 1973, and appears to have then taken a job at the VA. Along with two female cousins and her sister, Helen, she rented a small one-story white frame house in Ypsilanti Township. The neighborhood is a modest residential one.

Coincidentally, or so it appears, three of those who suffered suspicious arrests at the VA that summer lived close by.

Glenn Stout, who suffered arrests in late July and early August, lived just two blocks away; Benny Blaine, about four blocks away in the same direction; and Howard Leslie, the August 12 victim with only a broken elbow, across the nearest main street, perhaps as far as Blaine.

Had she known the victims before they came into the hospital?

Not as far as is publicly known.

It was just a coincidence, the FBI may have determined.

Once they reached the Ann Arbor stage of her life, the agents must have found it even easier to check on the nurse. But what they found was probably disappointing—at least in terms of solving the case quickly.

She seemed as correct and unassuming in her present life as she had in the past.

There wasn't much social life to speak of, as she had many responsibilities and duties and didn't seem to be the socializing kind. She was a practicing Catholic and churchgoer. As an immigrant, she was typically first-generation, prone to work hard and not make waves. And nobody, at least publicly, had anything bad to say about her.

"This girl has a good record," says Frank Burns, a day-shift ICU nurse and former Vietnam medic. "She comes with recommendations you wouldn't believe. And I know her and have seen her work. There's no one who fights for life more than she does."

The person (besides her cousins and sister) who has probably known her longer than anyone else in Ann Arbor is her landlord, Curt Branham, an auto company employee.

Referring to the entire household of his tenants, he told the *Free Press*: "I have never seen the girls take a drink. I have never seen them smoke a cigarette ... To my knowledge, none ... has a boyfriend ... They keep an immaculate house. There's just never been a problem with them. I just hold the highest esteem for them."

So high is his esteem, he added, that he sometimes entrusts the overnight care of his twelve-year-old only son to Narciso, and will continue to do so in spite of the investigation. She can't be guilty, he insisted.

Several young doctors at the hospital had similar feelings.

"She's very competent," said one upon hearing there was evidence against her, "understanding and sympathetic. I never saw anything about her character that would lead me to think she would do anything like this."

But the interns and residents only knew her on a professional level, the FBI could have concluded. And most of the older, permanent staff physicians didn't know her at all, and were probably more inclined to remain silent, or turn to the incriminating evidence, when asked by agents whether they thought she could have done it.

None of the believed victims, with the exception of McCrery, appears to have had anything derogatory to say about her. And even McCrery says that before his attack he was being treated "fine" by the ICU nurses.

One believed victim might even have praised her. Emmett Lutz, who suffered attacks in late July, volunteered that "the Filipinos were wonderful to me." But he could not be specific about which Filipinos he meant—at least not to non-governmental investigators.

Late in the investigation, James E. Thayer, a former patient of Narciso's, even wrote an impassioned letter which appears to be about and to her (he could not be reached), which the Ann Arbor *News* printed in its "Letters to the Editor" column.

"Two years ago I was in the VA Hospital for a very serious back operation ... In that time, I had great doctors and nurses ... One of these great and lovely girls was a foreign girl, many miles from her home. But to her, we were the men of the Army, Navy and Marine Corps who fought for, and sustained injury in defense of her country, in freeing that land from the Japanese.

"The evenings after my operation were very painful ones, and I found it very hard to sleep as I was in a body cast. Not only was there pain, but the uncomfortable cast kept me awake many nights. This girl would come to my bedside and ask if I was all right, if I needed anything, light a cigarette for me, get me a glass of water, bathe my forehead and talk with me.

Nothing was too great a task ... Many a night only her cheerful talk, and her being there, brought me through a very lonely and terrifying experience.

"I can only speak for myself, but I feel sure that many of these patients you cared for with compassion and understanding, will join me in a prayer ... that your ordeal will soon be over ... Good luck, and God bless you ... P.I. Narciso, R.N."

Youngsters, especially, appear to be her friends. It can be assumed that since she frequently cared for her landlord's son he enjoyed her company. And a young neighbor across the street, Kevin Smith, fifteen, was quoted by the Ypsilanti *Press* as saying he regularly went to her house for barbecues, "or just shooting baskets in the yard." She's "really nice," and "jokes a lot," Kevin told the reporter. And the basketball hoop—not something the Filipino girls would likely use—was apparently constructed for the neighborhood children.

Narciso had been at the VA approximately a year and a half when it appears (the hospital won't even divulge that information) she started working in its ICU. That would have been sometime in the spring of 1975, shortly before the hospital's arrest and death rates began to rise. The FBI probably viewed this with suspicion.

But some nurses say she was "rotated" to the ICU precisely because she was good at her job.

During the 1975 Christmas holidays, a visitor drove up and found Narciso parked in her driveway, the motor in her brown and tan late-model car idling. Apparently she had just arrived from work, where, since sometime after the investigation started, she'd been put in a non-patient position. The visitor identified himself as a writer from Florida and said he'd like to ask some questions. She declined courteously, saying her lawyer had advised her not to. Then she asked, "How do you like the snow?" The friendly question took the visitor by surprise, and he explained he'd probably get used to it.

There was small talk for a few minutes, and then, politely, she excused herself and headed for the front screen door. A small red sign with a frosted white NOEL printed across it hung loosely in the door's aluminum frame.

Such was the enigma of the little Filipino: responsible, considerate, shy. But was it a veil hiding evil beneath?

It didn't appear so to the writer—at least not at that moment. But apparently the FBI that first week of the investigation was less impressed. For they appear to have questioned her at length. And by the week's end, with their force inside the hospital increased to approximately ten agents, including Ward, and with Narciso still insisting on her innocence, they learned more about the crime.

The ad-hoc doctors' committee had by this time finished its deliberations. And the bureau itself, not wanting to rely solely on what the doctors said, had brought in professional data gatherers from Detroit. One or both of the two came up with the following additional seemingly incriminating facts:

An examination of all the suspicious codes revealed that Narciso had been at practically all the resuscitations and attempted resuscitations of the suspected victims. She had discovered one of the most suspicious arrests—Oelberg's—and possibly others. And she had even been filling in for someone else when the only suspicious early shift—8 A.M. to 4 P.M.—arrest had occurred. (It is not known exactly which arrest that was.)

In addition, something else interesting, as far as some of the agents were concerned, was discovered. Leonora

Perez, one of the other Filipinos, was found to have been at a lot of the codes too—not as many as Narciso, but a large number.

The two women protested, and rightfully so, that it was perfectly normal for them to have been at so many codes. As ICU nurses, it was their job to respond to emergencies. They were among the most highly trained on the shift, which itself was greatly understaffed, and it was their duty and obligation to respond.

What other incriminating facts, if any, the agents learned is not known. But the unexpected information about Perez began to intrigue some investigators. "Were the two in cahoots?" one official investigator says several started to wonder.

The evidence against Narciso was largely circumstantial. The evidence against Perez was hardly even that. And it appears the majority of agents only felt that she was a "material witness"—that is, a person with firsthand knowledge of some of the suspected attacks, but not necessarily with any active part in them.

But besides that, some of the agents were not satisfied with the answers they were receiving from the nurses—not only from Narciso or Perez, but other night-shift ICU staffers as well. They began, it appears, to suspect that lies were being told, or that certain vital pieces of information were being left out. (The nurses, for their part, say they cooperated, but started being harassed.) So in what seems to have been an investigative move (the results of the procedure, it appears, will not be admissible in court), the agents decided to ask the four or five ICU nurses to take polygraphs: lie-detector tests.

Little is known about the tests, but certain information has surfaced. Bonnie Bates Weston, of Ann Arbor, was one of the nurses asked. She, it developed, was the monitoring nurse in the CCU when McCrery had his suspicious arrest. They felt she should have seen something pertinent. But she maintained she hadn't. In her version, it has been reported, no one was around when she noticed McCrery starting to have difficulty. Then doctors rushed to him and began the resuscitation.

Weston may have refused to take the test once or twice, but eventually, it appears, she submitted. She failed at least one of the tests, says a Ypsilanti *Press* story, but "her attorneys ... say the tests were conducted improperly. For example, they say FBI agents were present during the tests—a violation of normal procedures." The test was used "as a method of intimidation," adds the *Press*, "not a means of determining whether Mrs. Weston was being truthful." Apparently the agents wanted her to have seen somebody beside McCrery's bed just before he began suffocating.

It seems equally certain that Narciso and Perez took the tests. Official investigators and their own lawyer— Perez also eventually hired O'Brien—say so. Exactly what happened, however, is unclear.

O'Brien says: "I've never been told what the results were. I know that on at least a couple of occasions 'P.I.' was asked to submit to a polygraph and voluntarily did so. The first time they were unable to conclude the test, I think, because there were too many people present. And the second time the test was given I have no idea what the results were."

But one FBI agent, says O'Brien, "told me the tests were inconclusive. And he indicated to me that both our clients, in particular 'P.I.', seemed nervous and was unresponsive even with such questions as 'Do you drink water?' And even though they said 'Yes' to that question, the machine was registering deceptive. And so he said that in his judgment they were just frightened by all this. Plus, there might have been some language barrier."

"Whether his analysis is correct I don't know."

Official investigators tell a similar story—except for one major part. The suspicions of some of the agents increased when they noted the nervousness. Some felt the results were something more than inconclusive: they were incriminating.

Why, if that report is correct, all the agents would not accept nervousness as a normal reaction to being charged with a mass murder—especially from women who are aliens and who may have been subjected to stressful interrogations—is known only to those who were there. But the final result of the testing appears to have been that more suspicion was directed toward the two nurses.

Around this time, it appears, the FBI also went to Dr. Derek H. Miller, professor of psychiatry at the University of Michigan and an authority on criminal personality. From England, Miller has a long list of credits in his résumé. They asked him to draw up a probable profile of the killer based on information they would provide. What Miller returned was a four-page report heavily emphasizing a person "sophisticated in pharmacology," "isolated" socially, and who was very probably an "angry" nurse.

Even before the FBI approached him, says Miller, he'd already guessed that the killer was probably a nurse. It's an odd phenomenon, he explains, that while patients usually always remember when their doctors come by to visit them, they seldom remember when the nurses do. "Nurses can move in and out without the slightest notice." Considering the large number of attacks, he says, it appeared obvious that only a nurse could have made them and not have been seen.

While Narciso didn't seem to be "angry," agents who wanted to might possibly have construed that her unmarried status and seeming lack of boy friends put her in the socially isolated category.

In addition, the FBI had, with the aid of the additional data about the murders they'd recently received, furnished Miller with the following statistical observation: with some 30 per cent of the hospital population black, only one of the suspected victims—Oulds, the retired coal miner from Flint—was a Negro.

One of the things this possibly meant, wrote Miller, was that the offender "identifies with 'underprivileged' blacks."

Filipinos were a minority group and might identify with other minorities, the FBI could have reasoned.

It might be incorrect to put so much emphasis on a psychiatric profile that the FBI may simply have filed, but while it appears that Perez at this time was still only being regarded as a material witness (she was married and had a child and at least one agent couldn't see "how anyone like that could have done such a thing"), the case against "P.I." seemed to be building.

Chapter 15

Even though it looked bad for Narciso, not every agent, in the beginning, was convinced she'd done it. In fact, some were inclined to think that, despite the evidence, it was more probable that the killer was a man.

The crime was so brazen, so sinister, a man seemed more likely. And, in fact, they had several leads that pointed to men.

Almost from the moment the investigation began, Loesch, the Vietnam veteran with the self-inflicted gunshot wound, had been claiming that he'd seen his attacker.

It was a white man, about 5'10" tall, he told Jim Schutze of the Detroit *Free Press* in an exceptional interview that appeared in newspapers across the country. It was just before he'd gone limp on August 15: "I felt a pain in my IV," he told Schutze, who surmounted authorities' orders of no interviews with patient-victims by posing as a friend on the phone. "I rolled over and looked. I saw a male going out the door. I just saw the back end."

Two of Benny Blaine's family members—Mary Prater and Betty Barnett—say that on August 12, when Benny had suffered his second suspicious attack, they'd seen a "tall" man in a "green doctor's coat," with a beard and possibly a mustache, come running out of the ICU just about the time the first Code 7 bulb lit up.

At first consideration, investigators probably felt the man's presence could be explained by saying he was a doctor involved in the ensuing resuscitation. But on second thought, that didn't fit.

The first code that night, which was on Blaine, was inside the ICU. So no doctors should have been running out.

The idea that the doctor must have been hurrying to get something needed in the resuscitation also didn't fit. The ICU was one of the few places in the hospital that summer where resuscitation equipment, always needed there, was usually in plentiful supply.

Finally, even if the equipment wasn't there, the two women said the man, who had a "black bag" in his hand, and nearly knocked them down with a gruff "Get out of the way," went straight for the closest stairs outside the ICU and quickly descended out of view.

This, it appears, would not have been the course of anyone legitimately involved in the first resuscitation. For a closer and more convenient set of doors leading to stairs was located inside the ICU itself.

A variety of the early leads pointing to males are only known in bits and pieces.

It appears that a young doctor was viewed suspiciously for a while. This coincided with the initial theory of some who noted that the suspicious arrests came right at the time when a new increment of medical students and residents had rotated into the hospital, and considered this more than coincidence. A deranged medical student sounded plausible—especially to the older, permanent staff.

The hunt for a "tall, bushy-haired man with glasses," or someone with some of these identifying features, is recalled by several hospital officials. In lesser degree, so is the search for a "black"; for a "former employee," who suddenly showed up back in the hospital; and even for a "custodian," seen "suspiciously looking over the shoulders of medical personnel."

But none of these leads—Loesch's, the Blaine family's, the various others—appears to have led to anything substantial. Whether or not the agents pursued them as diligently as they should have or whether the leads simply led to dead ends is not known.

By the end of the second week of the investigation, the FBI had enlarged its forces to approximately twenty men. They had swept through the hospital gathering up every item they felt might aid them in their search, and ensconced themselves in the north wing of the hospital's fifth floor. A sign on the wing's entrance doors said: AREA CLOSED. NO ADMITTANCE. Not even fifth-floor doctors were allowed without an escort.

Inside, agents set about poring over files and other pertinent papers, and conducting interviews. The Detroit data gatherers were probably utilized. Questioning was usually conducted with a staff doctor present to interpret the "medicalese." Even so, the technicalities were time-consuming and bogged down the investigation. "I've had to have a crash course in medicine just to stay even," one agent is quoted as saying.

But the FBI appears to have wanted to run it their way—not anybody else's. "They just took my observations and didn't give me any feedback," was the way one permanent staff physician described his interviews.

Adjoining the interview rooms, agents probably sifted what had been collected. Information was indexed and cross-indexed. The hope was to find a common denominator, any fact that would emerge as recurring, and thereby point in a single direction. Charts and graphs were constructed. One gets visions of morning blackboard briefings on the progress. However, few new leads developed. Everything continued to point back to the ICU.

It is estimated that by the time they were through, the agents had interviewed four hundred of the hospital's approximately one thousand employees. The bulk of the interviews were with those who worked on the late shift or had a free run of the hospital.

Cables were sent to FBI offices across the country asking other agents to check backgrounds of various VA staffers. The purpose was to find one who had worked at another hospital that might have experienced a similar string of mysterious deaths, or any problems whatsoever, because the agents were advised by psychiatrists that the maniac should have a history of at least petty crime.

In the course of such detective work, at least four other hospitals around the nation were found to have had unexplained deaths.

Almost immediately in the investigation, New Jersey authorities, who ten years before had probed thirteen mysterious deaths possibly involving curare, called Ann Arbor to get details of the Michigan crime. As a result, the former inquiry, which had been at Riverdell Hospital in Oradell, New Jersey, was reopened, and eventually an Englewood Cliffs surgeon, Dr. Mario Jascalevich, was indicted in five of the suspected murders.

Only a year before, in Marion, Illinois, Marion Memorial Hospital had been the scene of eight suspicious poisoning "accidents." With the publicity for the VA murders at full height, authorities there declared that the incidents were probably murder attempts. Stories from Marion told of emergency-room patients receiving what they thought were pain-relieving shots for minor injuries and then suddenly losing all control, falling back in suffocating spasms.

Also only a year before, a young male employee of Petersburg General Hospital, Petersburg, Virginia, was convicted of killing one of the hospital's cardiac patients with an injection of lidocaine, a drug which stops the heart. There were five other mysterious deaths at the hospital.

Agents must have wondered how many deaths at other hospitals around the country—if not at the Ann Arbor VA itself—were actually murder. But none of these, including a fourth string of possible drug deaths at an unnamed California hospital, so far as is known, provided any link to the Ann Arbor VA.

With the exception of McCrery, even interviews with the suspected VA victims were unproductive. Almost to a man, they were either groggy, sleeping, or turned the other way when they received their paralyzing shots. It must have been frustrating. Lutz said he felt "just like a lump of fruit" during his arrests. But he couldn't remember any more about them. Howard Leslie, who was only in for a broken elbow, had a total blank for almost an hour and a half before his attack.

Had the attacks been so horrible that the victims had shut them out of their memories? Agents must have wondered.

Then, around September, it appears, the FBI became aware of a major problem emerging in their case.

Before his respiratory arrest, McCrery had been scheduled for open-heart surgery. The operation was major and there were many complications that could ensue. It is not known how much the FBI was briefed on these complications, or what they decided if they were. But on August 20, the body shop owner left the

VA for the University of Michigan hospital, and August 22 the surgery was performed.

Medically, McCrery seems to have come through the operation well. Six weeks following it he was back home and watching football games. But, according to the FBI, he had developed a psychological problem. He was confused if not totally amnesiac about the days between his believed Pavulon attack and his surgery. This was crucial because much of what he had testified to in those few days was central to the government's case against "P.I."

Suddenly, he did not recall the nickname that others say he confirmed at least several times. Eventually it became apparent that he was identifying Perez as the nurse who had given him the paralyzing shot, and not "P.I." He himself insisted that he was perfectly sure of who it was, but that the FBI was mixed up about what he had said.

What had happened? Was it all a ruse? Had McCrery been lying all the time?

Not likely, the FBI and government prosecutors decided. You don't make up stories when you've just nearly lost your life. More likely, they felt, McCrery had suffered a psychological problem due to his surgery—a "memory loss" or "confusion," they were advised by his doctors. And, sure enough, when they went through the medical literature on the subject they found ample evidence that this could be the case.

Before such traumatic surgery as open-heart, postoperative psychological complications were rare. But since the introduction of new heart surgery techniques in about 1950 the incidence had been rising, especially among closed- and open-heart patients. (Closed-heart operations are those involving the heart but not opening it.) Indeed, among open-heart patients the figure, according to experts, was over 50 per cent.

According to Dr. Richard S. Blacher, writing in the October 16, 1972, issue of the *Journal of the American Medical Association* (JAMA), post-operative "psychosis" in open-heart patients includes confusion, paranoia, hallucinations, delusions and "loss of memory." One of the primary reasons for this, he writes, is that unlike an appendectomy or even a major operation such as a liver transplant, open-heart surgery involves possible damage to man's "historically and emotionally" most vital organ.

The sense of "awe" about the operation, he writes, is almost unbelievable. "It is almost unbearable for most patients to conceive of their hearts being incised ... One young man described vividly how he had worried little before his valve replacement. 'But after a few days, I began to realize what they'd done to me, opening my heart and all, and wow! I let myself realize what I'd gone through and became unbelievably frightened.'"

In open-heart, the blood is rerouted from the organ and circulated by means of a huge "heart-lung" machine, which pumps and oxygenates it. This allows surgeons, who have opened the chest, to repair the heart. Bloodless chambers can be entered, valves replaced. The machine keeps the patient alive.

There appears to be a direct relationship between the amount of time on the machine and the amount and degree of post-operative psychosis, speculates Blacher.

It is not known how long McCrery was on the "pump." But he himself says that "for days" following his surgery "I didn't know what was happening." He didn't recognize his wife, and told her he saw attacking "dragonflies." But after about a week, he says, these problems had disappeared. He was back to what he considered normal, and remembered just about everything up to and including his attack.

Given the added trauma of a near fatal murder attempt just prior to his surgery, it's probable that McCrery did experience "retrograde amnesia," or, at least, some form of "post-pump psychosis," as it's also sometimes called. But as early as three weeks into his recovery he was saying that it wasn't Narciso who had given him the shot. She may have been in the room, he said, but it was another Filipino (later, if not at that time, identified as Perez) who had made the attack.

This was a serious blow to the prosecution's case. McCrery was the only eyewitness they had, and now he was changing his story. It meant that the case against Narciso was suddenly only circumstantial. They had substantial testimony from others that McCrery had identified Narciso. But would a jury believe a witness who had switched his story? And although it's not certain why the FBI didn't regard the switch as useful in their burgeoning case against Perez, it doesn't appear they did. "The first version fit better," says one insider.

In any event, investigators saw their case deteriorating. All other leads had fizzled and they had been unable to turn up any new ones. In addition, it had been nearly a month since the investigation had begun, and the hospital administration—and probably Washington too—was calling for an end to the near siege conditions the institution had been operating under.

Since the first day, in addition to the limitation of admissions, which necessitated turning away sick veterans, doctors had been required to sign in at a security table upon every visit to the ICU. There were rigid new procedures governing the requisition of drugs, and regulations forbidding IV injections without at least one other person present.

By mid-September, several more suspected victims had died, Blaine and Oelberg among them, raising the death toll still higher, and putting even more pressure on the agents to come up with the killer.

Still hoping for a quick end to the case, they decided to go back one more time and try to force a confession out of Narciso. What happened at the session, as in all other crucial sessions conducted by the FBI, is known only to the participants and those they've chosen to discuss it with. The following is an unofficial account:

The questioning lasted six hours. Narciso's lawyer, O'Brien, says his client told him that agents came to her house around noon of a September day and told her to be at the hospital at 2 P.M. Once there, a nonstop grilling began.

According to O'Brien, who has notes given to him by his client shortly after the questioning, the agents first tried to coax her into a confession by saying that maybe it was all a mistake. " 'You just wanted to relax' " the victim, she wrote they said to her. But " 'you gave him too much.' "

But then, with the FBI getting nowhere, says O'Brien, his client wrote, "they became harsh," and said it was intentional. " 'You're in a dilemma,' " they said. " 'You're twenty-nine and look at your life. It's over. You can confess and we'll rehabilitate you.' "

"I felt terrible," Narciso wrote. "These people were stronger. They were accusing me. They said 'All the facts we've gathered point to you and we want to help you . . . But you're in a dilemma. The jury [members] aren't stupid. They will prove you guilty.'

"They said don't be a 'Joan of Arc. Do you want us to dig up bodies to prove you're the one giving the Pavulon?' I asked them 'If you were in my shoes, would you answer yes to things you hadn't done? One of them said, 'You're abnormal. You ask more questions than you're asked.'"

Three times during the interrogation, says O'Brien, Narciso asked to leave, but each time was denied permission.

Toward the end, he says, the agents said something like "You're a woman of strong Catholic beliefs. Well, you'd better go light a novena candle because you're going to need it." Narciso took this as an insult, says O'Brien. It was bringing her religion into the probe. She became upset.

It was 8 P.M. before the grilling ended, he says, and his client emerged in tears.

The FBI does not deny that the marathon interrogation took place. In fact, the authorities, while saying whatever tactics they used were justified, offered to apologize for the session.

But in the FBI version, Narciso was "tough"—not crying—during the ordeal. And this, they say, solidified at least the interrogators' belief that she was the kind of person who could have committed the murders.

Which version is right? The answer may never be known.

But a short time afterward, some of the ICU nurses went public with their grievances.

A September 27 story in the Ypsilanti *Press* blared: VA NURSES QUIT OVER FBI "HARASSMENT." Other newspapers, TV and radio stations soon carried their own versions. Narciso and Perez were not among the quitters. But it was clear that the action was taken mostly on their behalf.

The Ypsi article said between two and five nurses had handed in their resignations. Charges included late-night visits to nurses' homes, shining lights in their faces, pounding fists on tables, shouting, and "pitting" one girl against another. "You have to understand this is a very intensive investigation," Gary Calhoun was quoted as telling the reporter.

Asked if she was "concerned that FBI agents were too tough or too persistent," Gloria Nunley, head of the VA's nursing department, replied: "The FBI is an agency of the government which came in to help in an assertive way to determine what happened here ... I have discussed their approach to the interviews with management and members of the investigation team and they assured me they were using appropriate tactics although in some instances it might seem different than that."

Most employees at the hospital felt the FBI had conducted themselves admirably.

It should be noted that throughout all the heavy questioning neither Narciso or Perez had been represented by counsel; it was shortly after the six-hour session that they both hired O'Brien.

Chapter 16

Sometime at the end of September, the FBI completed its initial investigation. Agents dismantled the fifth-floor headquarters and carted off stacks of papers and charts they had accumulated, depositing résumés, if not complete copies, in the downtown Detroit offices of Assistant U. S. Attorney Delonis.

By this time, it appears, a computer study had further profiled the crime. Programming respiratory arrest data from the VA for an entire year, a team headed by Dr. Jeoffrey K. Stross, an assistant director at the University of Michigan's Department of Postgraduate Medicine, determined that twenty of the approximately fifty breathing failures between July 1 and August 15 were in a "high suspicion" category—that is, "unexpected and not compatible with the natural history of the patient's disease" or "the attending physician's evaluation of [that] disease."

Compared to previously determined figures, this meant that the number of officially designated victims of the attacks was rising.

And so was the official death toll.

The computer showed that six of those who had suffered the twenty "highly suspicious" arrests had died. This too was up from the one or two "probables" the earlier ad-hoc committee had found.

But the number of *patients* suffering the computer-designated arrests doesn't appear to have been twenty. Several on the list had experienced more than one arrest, possibly two or three.

(The Ann Arbor *News* reported that the twenty "highly suspicious" arrests involved only fifteen patients. Stross himself refused to discuss the statistics.)

These multiple arrests suffered by some of the believed victims had the FBI and Delonis wondering: had the killer returned to "finish off" victims? Had he or she "scouted" patients? Or was it just that certain circumstances, such as location of beds, provided more opportunity for attack?

The first possibility suggested a real and monstrous savagery in the killer. The second meant the multiple attacks resulted only from circumstance—a patient being in a particular place at a particular time.

Whatever the meaning of the multiple arrests, the computer was more suggestive about another finding: many of the "highly suspicious" arrests (as previously suspected) had indeed come in "clusters," Stross, in a speech to a specially invited audience of doctors, later revealed. This, he said, was at variance with the sporadic and unconnected manner in which "natural" arrests had occurred.

It suggested the killer would go on grim rampages, attacking groups of helpless patients whose beds were close together—as apparently had happened on the nights of August 12 and 14.

Obviously the killer had gone berserk on the afternoon of August 15 when there were two clusters of arrests in quick succession: three in the ICU and two on a floor above. Moreover, five of the twenty computer-designated "highly suspicious" arrests occurred *outside* the ICU, and were preceded by what the data determined were "natural" arrests, or arrests of "low" or "no" suspicion.

This meant, theorized Stross, that the killer sometimes used natural arrests outside the ICU as vehicles from which to launch strikes in the hospital's less-guarded areas.

"It is postulated that the cardiac-arrest team was called to a floor for an arrest, and during the resuscitation efforts, a series of assaults were made on patients in surrounding rooms, either across the hall or next door," Stross wrote.

This pattern fits what appears to have happened on several of the suspect nights. On August 12, Drs. Penner and Weber had been called to resuscitate Fenton Borst, and midway in the procedure had been suddenly notified that Howard Leslie, a relatively healthy patient in the room next door, was in arrest. On August 14, almost identical episodes had been reported by Drs. Zibrak and Mcleod concerning patients Green and Oelberg.

The killer's probable "MO"—method of operation—was emerging from the data. And in many of the computer-brought-to-mind incidents, as the discovery of Oelberg on the fourteenth, it was a nurse who had done the "discovering."

The circumstantial case, it appears, continued to build against ICU nurses. But reviewing the case so far accumulated, there were still major hurdles that Delonis (a large man of thirty-four, who at one time wanted to be a priest) had to surmount before hoping to get an indictment against any nurses—especially Narciso, even though at that time she was the prime, if not the only real, suspect.

To begin with, no clear-cut motive had surfaced.

From the beginning of the investigation, agents had repeatedly heard that hospital personnel—especially the ICU nurses—were distraught if not angered by the VA's help shortage. Several times nurses had formally protested. In one of the most overt protests, fifty-seven nurses from several departments had signed a petition demanding more help be hired. Their overtime hours were excessive, with no time off, the nurses charged. Some even threatened to quit.

Could this have been the motive for the attacks, some investigators began wondering. Could, in the demented minds of a few, the killings have been the ultimate protest to the administration to signal that the situation had to be changed?

At first, it appears, this theory was discounted by Delonis and the agents. It just didn't seem possible that so comparatively minor a problem (although believed crucial in saving lives by some of the nurses) could have provoked so ghastly a solution. But as the weeks advanced, with no other motive materializing, and as the evidences of the nurses' strong feelings about the shortage piled up, the prosecutors, it appears, began to look at it seriously.

Mercy killing had to be ruled out because a sizable number of the victims had not been seriously ill.

For a while, investigators speculated that perhaps the killer was like some arsonists and brought on the arrests to observe the fight for life. But at least some of the patients were asleep or in stupors when struck, thus eliminating any real observable suffering. And others in remote rooms and wards were never even resuscitated, dying unseen. In addition, it had been reported, the computer did not find any one employee at all the suspicious codes. This, too, argued against a "watcher."

Sometime during the investigation, someone remembered that among the many victims of Richard Speck's

1966 mass murder of nursing students in a Chicago apartment house there had been Filipinos. In fact, the lone survivor and only witness to the murders had been a Filipino.

Perez had lived in Chicago at one time, it had been determined. And, for a while, there must have been some scrambling for additional facts. But no link between the two crimes was ever established, according to Delonis, who later commented on it in response to press inquiries.

Returning to their records, the investigators pondered. All the victims were men, which, given the ratio of male to female patients in the hospital, was to be expected. They ranged in age from their late twenties to early eighties, and had served in all the major American conflicts of the century: World Wars I and II, Korea and Vietnam. There was no shared characteristic in their personal or occupational lives, except for their common war experience.

Since there just wasn't anything else suggesting a motive, Delonis, it appears, decided the nursing shortage and resultant overworking of the staff would have to suffice—at least until something more substantial came along.

The next major problem was even more crucial.

Although investigators had much data and many opinions indicating crimes had been committed, they had little physical evidence, such as the syringes used, with which to prove it.

In early September the tests on fluids taken from the August 15 victims had come in. They were positive (although, for a while, there was worry they weren't conclusive enough). The labs said the urine taken from McCrery and Loesch—the only two victims who were catheterized that afternoon when crime was first suspected—reacted just as it should have if Pavulon was present. Combined with the clinical impressions of the doctors at the arrest scenes, the nerve stimulator tests and the quick recoveries each of the victims had made when given the antidote, Delonis and his staff would probably be able to prove that the three had been poisoned with the drug since none was supposed to have been receiving it.

But, it appears, they had little, if any, such evidence relating to the other suspected victims—apparently only clinical impressions and analyses of the patients' records.

The computer had determined that fourteen of the twenty "highly suspicious" arrests had involved "extreme flaccidity"—the telltale sign of a muscle relaxer. And the victims in a majority of those arrests had recovered in the time period suggestive of a Pavulon dose—approximately three and three quarters hours.

But that was not *physical* evidence.

The major reason the prosecutors appeared to have this dearth of evidence is that Pavulon, like many other such drugs, passes through the body quickly. Once administered, roughly half the dose is secreted through the urine in the first twenty-four hours. The rest, according to pharmacologists, is gone in a matter of days.

Since the attacks had not been discovered as such until at least a month and a half after they'd started, most of the victims had already flushed the evidence down urinals and toilets—and those who hadn't were dead.

But somewhat ironically, those corpses, the darkest result of the crime, offered the prosecutors their best chance to recoup evidence, the experts told them.

Among the suspected murder victims, there were patients who'd died right at the times of their arrests. These patients had not had a chance to urinate, and, consequently, the drug might still be in their bodies.

As it was standard procedure routinely to examine all deaths at the VA, autopsies by unaware pathologists had probably emptied all the veins and bladders. And Pavulon (pancuronium) was an especially elusive drug to find. But given luck and a lot of hard work, the prosecutors were told, there was a chance that somewhere in the recesses of the corpses—perhaps in minor organs or in tissue to which Pavulon, for physiological reasons, might gravitate—they might just find the poison.

Among the experts advising the government was Dr. Bert N. La Du, head of the University of Michigan's Pharmacology Department. La Du, it turns out, was uniquely suited to give such advice. While serving as professor of pharmacology at New York University, he had been a prosecution witness in one of the few other murder cases involving a muscle-relaxer—the celebrated Dr. Carl Coppolino trial of the late 1960s.

Coppolino was charged with killing his wife with succinylcholine, a less potent muscle-relaxer, but one just as elusive and widely used. (It had been one of the drugs that at the beginning of the investigation doctors had thought might have been the VA murder drug.) Coppolino was convicted in the Naples, Florida, trial, and La Du was one of those who had helped find the drug in the wife's exhumed body.

It appears La Du was only approached for an opinion in the VA case. But make no mistake, he says he told agents, like finding the succinylcholine in Mrs. Coppolino, there would be some formidable obstacles to positively finding pancuronium.

For one thing, he said, the drug was so new that although technicians could find it in urine, no one yet knew how to detect it in human tissue—assuming it still was in the buried bodies. Pancuronium is one of the newest synthetic curares, the prosecutors were told.

Developed for its strength and speed, it didn't come into general use until the 1960s. Although its commercial manufacturers had subjected it to a variety of needed tests, they had not yet devised ways to detect it in decomposed human flesh. Totally new tests would have to be developed. It could take months.

Moreover, pancuronium was one of those drugs that did not "take well" to tissue. There was a strong chance that with the autopsies and other circumstances, the drug had completely vanished. If the prosecutors embarked on such a search, the experts advised, they'd have to be prepared for disappointment.

There probably wasn't much debate over what to do. As beset with problems as the search might be, and despite the potential useless cost to taxpayers should the search fail, it was the prosecution's only chance of coming up with indisputable evidence that murder had been committed.

They wanted such evidence.

Sometime in September, it appears, the decision was made to go ahead and begin seeking permissions from the suspected victims' families for exhumation of the bodies.

But which of the families to approach?

Delonis, it seems certain, now had a list of probable murder victims that could have had as many as ten names on it. But victims like Benny Blaine or Adam Oelberg wouldn't do. Both had died weeks after their attacks and consequently would have already passed the Pavulon from their systems before expiring.

No, the prosecutors had been told, only in those who had died during or immediately following a suspect arrest could they hope to find the drug.

Probably after much deliberation, Delonis and his staff settled on four former patients as most likely to yield the desired results: Green, Oulds and Ogle from the August 14 attacks; and Herman, the double amputee who died July 30. There's a possibility more might have been exhumed. But these four are all that have become publicly known.

On October 2, in a cold dawn chill, a large yellow earthmover began plunging its scooped shovel into the neatly packed dirt of Mt. Ever-Rest Cemetery, Kalamazoo, Michigan. Six feet down, Joseph Green's body lay interred. It was the third exhumation. Herman and Ogle had already been dug up. Oulds's body was to be removed from a Flint cemetery the next morning.

Two overcoated FBI agents stood on the far side of the grave. Delonis, his hands in his pockets, observed from its foot. Mrs. Bernice Green, Green's wife, is also in a picture of the exhumation that appeared in the Detroit *Free Press*. "I just want to be with the body before they close the casket again," she told a *Free Press* reporter. "You might think that's gruesome, but that's what I want." Later she said, "I went to see that everything was handled right."

Since her husband's death, Mrs. Green had received no official word from the hospital or investigators about what had happened. When the FBI had come asking her permission for the exhumation, she'd taken the opportunity to find out more. "They are looking for the poison," she told the reporter. "I mean that's the way I understand it. They don't tell you too much."

When the casket, buried August 18 (a month and a half before), was finally reached, it was lifted into a waiting gray hearse and driven away. Following it were agents in a station wagon "loaded with containers for the tissue samples," and Mrs. Green in a second car. "They took it to a funeral parlor about two miles away," she says. "I didn't see what was done, but they told me they'd taken a slice from each organ."

A "decoy" hearse had gone elsewhere to throw the press off, she says.

Following all the exhumations, the tissue samples were sent to the FBI lab in Washington, and possibly elsewhere, so the difficult work could begin. Investigators then turned to their final major problem—the lack of witnesses to the crime.

As far as can be determined, by early October, the only eyewitness investigators had was McCrery. Out of all the surviving victims they knew of—possibly as many as fifteen—he was the only one who remembered seeing anything pertinent.

It was a unique situation. Usually in cases involving as many incidents as did the VA murders and murder attempts there was more than one witness. Certainly more firsthand knowledge of the crimes. The prosecutors had to wonder if special conditions were at work here—such as some of the victims simply blocking the experience out of their minds.

Whatever they wondered, they eventually hit on an idea: hypnotism could sometimes reactivate buried memories. Only recently, according to the Ypsi *Press*, "agents hypnotized friends of missing former Teamster boss Jimmy Hoffa [who had disappeared from Detroit July 30 and was the object of an intensive FBI hunt at the same time the VA case was unfolding] to see if they remembered whom he told them he was going to see the day he disappeared." Why couldn't it do some good for them?

Delonis says: "I did some legal research to see what had been done before. There were some interesting cases. One in Maryland involved an assault and rape—a brutal thing on a highway. The victim had blotted it out of her mind, but a hypnotist had had remarkable success in recapturing her memory. So there was a precedent."

But the procedure was unusual. It certainly was not totally accepted in the legal community. They would have to be extremely careful how they did it, says Delonis. There were certain rules and regulations to follow. They would have to find an eminently qualified hypnotist, and then they would have to ensure that what followed was as unchallengeable as possible. They were not, it appears, hoping to get whatever the sessions might reveal entered into evidence; but merely to help the patients revive memories and develop leads.

They must have done more research. Delonis says Washington "approved" the decision. Then, after a search for their specialist, they settled on Dr. Herbert Spiegel, associate clinical professor of psychiatry at the College of Physicians and Surgeons, Columbia University, New York City.

Unlike "stage hypnotists," Spiegel was a medical doctor and psychiatrist who used hypnosis as a clinical aid in treating patients. "His credentials showed he had everything it took," says Delonis. He had even been involved, as a defense witness, in one of the few cases where a conviction obtained by faulty hypnosis had been overturned. So not only was he expert in *how* to use hypnosis, says Delonis, he was expert in how *not* to use it.

Spiegel specializes in using his hypnotic skill to help patients stop smoking. Interviewed in his Manhattan office, he stressed that hypnosis is "disciplined concentration," rather than a "sleep" or dream state. The hypnotized person is simply able to recall imprinted memories that are unrecallable in the normal state of consciousness. He did not discuss a hypnotist's abilities to influence the actions of a subject, but said that in cases involving criminal matters, the key was in the questioning. Instead of asking, "Did so-and-so do this to you?" the question should be "What happened on such and such a date?" The subject should never be led, he said.

Having worked on a variety of criminal cases, Spiegel accepted the invitation by the Detroit prosecutors, and was told he would later be given a time and date to come.

The next problem was deciding which patients—and possibly non-patients—might be good subjects for hypnosis. It promised to be a lengthy and somewhat grueling affair for all those involved, and the prosecutors wanted to make the most of the time and participants they would have.

The government has remained silent about who took part. But interviews with some of the victims have revealed at least four of those involved, and two who were not. And several possible participants can be speculated upon.

Lutz, VanDenBerg and Neely from the late July attacks confirmed they took part, and so did Leslie from August 12. Not hypnotized were Gasmire and Richards, and possibly other victims. Gasmire, one of the oldest to be suspected of having suffered an attack, said the FBI had asked him, but "I went through enough without letting them make a guinea pig out of me." He turned them down. Richards, one of the eight August 12 arrests, said he was still too ill to participate.

Press reports have said McCrery and Loesch participated. And because McCrery's memory was so central to the case, and Loesch, too, had said he'd seen somebody near his bed at the time of one of his arrests, it's probable they did. As to who the others were—and there are indications there were others—one can only speculate. But there was reason for the prosecutors to want to hypnotize some of the ICU nurses, including Narciso and Perez, although it is not believed those two took part. (Several reports say they were asked but understandably declined.)

However, it's possible that some of the other ICU nurses might have undergone hypnotism, and so might some of the staff doctors, such as Lucy Goodenday, who had seen crucial events and might have welcomed clarification.

In any case, by mid-December, and after the grand jury had already begun considering evidence in the case, the prosecutors, hypnotist, victims and others were at last ready for the experiment.

As each person reported to the VA, where it had been decided the sessions would be held, the prosecutors, at least, had their fingers tightly crossed.

Chapter 17

It was December 16. In rooms somewhere near or at the top of the VA, several of the arrest victims had already been hypnotized. Now Richard Neely, the cancer patient who suffered an arrest the night of July 30, was sitting in a chair facing four interrogators: the hypnotist, Dr. Spiegel; and Special Agents Richard Guttlen, Daniel Russo and Pat Mullany. Perhaps five others, including prosecutor Delonis, were on the shadowy fringes.

The sessions with Neely promised to be the most controversial. In an October statement to the FBI, he had identified Narciso from a group of photos saying she and another Filipino nurse who was not pictured had visited him in his hospital room from "time to time." Although then he had remembered almost nothing about his arrest, the agents were particularly interested in what he was now recalling.

Bright lights illuminated Neely and his interrogators. The sessions were being video-taped so anyone questioning the procedure could see exactly what happened. But the atmosphere was relaxed, or at least the government was trying to make it appear so. That was the only way they could hope to achieve success. Pressure could ruin a session. They spoke calmly. Their sitting positions were casual. Whenever Neely had said something seemingly important they'd tried to hide their interest.

Neely had been "remembering" for perhaps fifteen minutes. He had just now taken his listeners back to his hospital room that fateful July 30, only moments prior to his near-fatal arrest. From official government sources and documents, and a taped interview with Neely, here is an abbreviated version of what actually followed:

His room was 462, Neely vividly remembered. It was approximately 10 P.M. He was wearing pajamas, and was propped up by pillows on his bed. IV lines ran into his right arm. A dim light from the hallway cast shadows in the room, but it was still "dark" and "real quiet." Suddenly he saw himself "gasping" for breath and vigorously shaking an aluminum guard rail on the side of the bed.

"What's the matter?" asked one of the agents.

"Just seems like I was trying to get my breath and I couldn't hardly do it. So I shook the bed hard for a nurse."

"Why are you shaking it?" another inquired.

"I'm mad, I'm hollering 'Hey, nurse. Hey, nurse!'"

"Are your eyes open?" asked Dr. Spiegel.

"Yes, halfway open ... I could hold 'em about halfway open because they were going shut."

"Was there anybody near you?"

"No. No, I don't see nobody."

"Well, why are you mad?"

"Because I hollered once ... twice. And she didn't come. What the hell kind of a place is this. What do you have to do to get a nurse?"

"Can you see the room?" said Spiegel.

"Yeah, I guess it was that little room."
"Can you see anybody in it?"
"No."
"Eyes open?"
"Yeah."
"Now look around before you call the nurse, Dick," an agent said. "Do you see that on your screen?"
"Yeah."
"Do you see the needles—see the [IV] needles in your arm?"
"Yeah."
"What else?"
"It seems like somebody was there with me. Seems like somebody was moving."

The attention of those in the room must have suddenly heightened. This, it appears, was the first time any hypnotized victim had indicated he might have seen the assailant.

"You say it seems like somebody was moving, Dick?" said Spiegel. "On which side does this movement take place?"
"All on the right side."
"What is the movement?" asked an agent.
"It seems like it was somebody—that's what it seems like."
"Look on your screen, Dick," said the agent. "Try and focus clearly. Does it appear to be a man or woman?"
"It seems like it's a man."
"Any colors?" said Spiegel.
"I can't see it," answered Neely. "I saw 'em come in my room there a few times. They had me kind of wondering."
"What colors do you see?" repeated Spiegel.
"Black," said Neely.
"Black?"

"That's the color of the person that was in there," said Neely.

"Can you see the black person coming into the room?" asked an agent.

"Not that particular night. Not when I hollered for the nurse."

"No," says the agent, forgetting himself a bit. "I'm talking about *now*—a minute before you called the nurse."

"Oh," says Neely. "No."

Apparently he was recalling another night.

Spiegel returned to the lead.

"Dick, you have that movement there. What is that movement you're seeing on your right?"

"I don't know . . . I thought it was somebody."

"Now on your screen, when you say you thought it was somebody. Try and focus in on who you thought it was . . . Is it big? Small? Moving? Still?"

Previously, agents had established that two nurses, one male and one female, known to Neely only as "Pancho" and "Nancy," had been visiting him just prior to his arrest. Moments later, when they said they'd heard Neely shaking his bed and calling for help, they'd rushed back from a break they were taking nearby, and found him "turning blue." Checking it out, the FBI, it appears, had accepted the story, and did not believe Pancho or Nancy was criminally involved in the arrest. Pancho was one of those Neely would now refer to. And Nancy, too, would soon come up.

"All I know is Pancho wouldn't do anything like that," Neely responded. "That could not have been Pancho. But everyone I think of . . . they wouldn't do nothing like that. It couldn't have been Bill. Debbie and all the nurses, they wouldn't do nothing like that . . ."

"What'd they do?" asked an agent.

"Well, they did something to knock me out one night. But I just hardly believe any of them could do anything like that."

"On your screen," said an agent, "can you see who would do something like that?"

"I kind of hate to say because there's been so much talk about it, that I . . . There's nothing . . . not enough, not enough . . ."

"Just tell us what you see."

"That one Filipino girl . . ."

"Describe."

"She comes in my room. Don't get a bit friendly. Everything she says is yes, no. That's about what she'd say. Yes. No. But the other little Filipino girl, she was friendly. She'd talk. She'd stay right there till I'd take my pill and make sure I'd take it. But the other one is kind of snotty. But she does things like that . . . And there's not enough, uh, proof, or anything in what I'm saying. Shouldn't even say anything about her."

"You just tell us what's on your screen . . . What do you see in the background?"

"Nancy."

"When? Before you had trouble?"

"Yeah—she's checking tubes."

"How do you feel?"

"Good . . . She straightened up the bed . . . She and Pancho leave the room. Then it's dark . . . Then I'm shaking the bed."

"How long after they left are you shaking the bed?"

"Not five minutes later."

"You don't see anything else from the time they left to the time you started shaking the bed?"

"No."

"Try and focus on Nancy and the other leaving. See anything? Any movement? Can you see any movement before you go to sleep?"

"No. I can't see nothing moving and nobody. They ran."

"Now, on your screen, go to the first point that you feel uncomfortable. What's on your screen?"

"I just woke. I just couldn't breathe."

"Okay. On your screen. What do you see? How do you feel?"

"I wanted a nurse ... I was mad ... I couldn't get my breath."

"Any pain?"

"No. No pain because before they got me down to that other room [he was rushed to the ICU shortly after he was discovered] my hands and arms were paralyzed and my feet was all paralyzed. I couldn't move nothing, only my eyelids."

"Any sensation in either arm? [Some of the victims reported a stinging sensation when the Pavulon entered their veins.]"

"No. I remember I couldn't move my fingers, hands, arms ... not a toe or a foot."

"Now put yourself at the point when you first started to gasp," said an agent. "See any movement? Someone in your room? Someone going out?"

The reference to a Filipino must have excited some of the interrogators. It appears they were trying to get Neely to return to it without obviously leading him.

"Seems like the movement was there," replied Neely. "But they left ... I don't know, I don't really ... I couldn't really say who left. I don't know. I don't remember."

"How many do you see leaving?"

"Two."

"Is that when you gasped for breath?"

"Yeah, right. After they walked out I started to gasp for breath. And I didn't think they were very far away ... I thought they could easily hear me. But they didn't come back. They didn't come back and I hollered and hollered."

"Do you know their names?"

"I thought it was Nancy and Pancho. They followed each other out..."

At this point the interrogators called for a break. They had been on the verge, they probably felt, of hearing more that might intensify their case against the Filipinos. But Neely was wandering. They couldn't bring him back. And Nancy and Pancho had been crossed off as possible suspects. There was no evidence against them.

It had been an intense first session with Neely. Everyone headed outside for coffee.

It was probably half an hour later when they regathered in the rooms for Neely's second session. The questioners brought Neely back to a few moments after Pancho and Nancy had left his room.

"Okay," said an agent. "Now we want slow motion on your screen. Your eyes are open, right?"

"Yeah," said Neely.

"Are you looking around the room?"

"Yes."

"What happens next?"

"I can't breathe."

"Do you see anything?"

"No."

"Go back. Pancho and Nancy have just left. Concentrate on the door. See anyone come in?"

"No."

"Do you see any movement at all?" Spiegel asked.

"Yes, it seems like there's movement in there. That's why I got so mad when I had to holler for a nurse."

"You see movement now?" said an agent.

"Yeah, there must have been somebody else in there."

"Okay, now on your screen, listen to yourself hollering. What do you holler?"

"Nurse! Hey, nurse!"

"Did you do that once?"

"Two or three times," replies Neely.

"Now when you said this, was somebody there?"

"Seems like there was, but I still had to holler."

"Could you see a nurse?"

"No . . . I don't believe so."

"Look carefully."

"Yeah! Somebody! It seemed like there was somebody there but I still had to holler for a nurse and it made me awful mad."

"Okay," said an agent. "Look at the scenes just when you hollered. What do you see?"

"Well, it's sorta like . . . like maybe one, two or three could have been there. It seems like people was there but I had to holler for a nurse."

"Did you expect the person in your room to respond to your holler?"

"No, that's why I had to holler . . . I don't know whether I asked 'em or not."

"If they were there, Dick, can you describe these people?"

"Make it slow motion," said Spiegel. "Describe the movements and shapes you see."

"Seems like I don't know them, or else I didn't get a real good look at them."

"How tall are they? Same height?"

"If there was two or three, I don't think any of them was a tall man. But I ain't sure if there was anybody even in the room . . . But it seemed like I got mad because they wouldn't do something for me, so I had to holler for Nancy and Pancho."

"Go back," said an agent. "What made you mad?"

"Don't know . . . fell back in bed . . . then Nancy and Pancho came in and found me."

Through a few more questions and answers, Neely seemed confused—as if he was in the ICU. But then he said he was back in room 462 and he heard "somebody scuffling around. It was somebody gettin' their ass outa there in a hurry."

"Okay," said an agent, "one frame at a time. What did you see? What did you feel?"

"There were more people in my room after Nancy and Pancho left. There were more people in there."

"Before you started to feel uncomfortable and after Pancho and Nancy left?"

"Yeah, yes, there was. There had to be . . . because there was feet a-scuffling around."

"You're in 462 and there are feet scuffling around?"

"Yeah."

"What do you see?"

"It seems like there was two or three, but Pancho and Nancy would know."

"Look to your right [where his IVs were]," said an agent. "Is this where the activity is? The scuffling? The scuffling of the feet?"

"Yeah, down at the foot end of the bed and all around."

"Before or after your shortness of breath?"

"Before."

"Do you hear anybody say 'Hello, Mr. Neely' after Pancho and Nancy leave?"

"No."

"Okay. Now concentrate on your arm. What do you see? Take your time—slow motion."

"I can see . . . I shouldn't exactly tell that . . . say that on 'em."

"Say it," said Dr. Spiegel.

205

"That short colored fellow. You know I ain't got no proof of him doing anything."

Just before the second session, Neely had said he wanted to tell his questioners something he'd been afraid before to tell "because I might get somebody in trouble." Apparently unaware that he had mentioned a black man in the first session, he told of a "short, stocky colored fellow" coming into his room and "pulling" and "studying" his IVs for a long time. "I've often wondered what the hell he was doing in there like that?" But because Neely said this had not been on the night of his arrest, investigators had dropped it.

Now, however, they appeared interested.

"Describe what you see on your screen," said an agent, "slowly from the top."

"When I hollered they had to do some shuffling to get out of there."

"What do you see, Dick? Take your time. Tell us what's there. You have to tell us what's there because we can't see it."

"All I can see, all I can see," he said anxiously, "is me hanging on the side of that bed hollering for a nurse."

"Back up, back up," said an agent.

"You skipped two frames," said another.

"Very slowly," said the first. "Do you see the tubes? Do you see someone there?"

"It just seems like shadows," said Neely. "You know, like if you have someone pass you in the dark. Say two or three . . . together . . . You know what it is but you can't see them."

"Can you see the shadows?" said an agent. "Stop the frame. Is it getting brighter?"

"I hate to say what I see right now," answered Neely.

"Tell us . . . Tell us what you see."

"That Filipino girl and that colored fellow . . . Now why should I pick on them two?"

"Describe the girl," said an agent, "the Filipino girl."

"She's thin, stacked nice."

"How tall is she?"

"She might be five two, five four."

"What color is her hair?"

"Black."

"Is it short, medium or long?"

"Down about her shoulders."

Leonora Perez fit that description. (Of course, so might other Orientals.)

"Do you know her name?" asked an agent.

"Well, I always just call her doll. Both of 'em, I call 'em dolls. But I don't know either one of their names."

Here agents might have recalled Neely's earlier statements about Narciso and another Filipino visiting him from "time to time."

"Do you notice anything unusual about her facial features?"

The reason for this question is not clear. Was it simply to reveal Oriental features? Or was there something more specific they were looking for?

"Now I wonder," said Neely, "did she have a scar on her face somewhere . . . above her eye?"

"Wearing glasses?" said an agent.

"No."

"What about the black person?" asked another.

"The short, stocky fellow that comes in there? He was in my room two or three times . . ."

"Okay," interrupted the first agent, "but the nurse? What is *she* doing?"

"She never liked me very well," said Neely. "I don't believe I talked to her but a bit, but there was just something about her that she just couldn't get very friendly like the other one did."

"Are you saying something to her now?"

"Yeah, I always . . . I would say 'Hi, doll. How are you this evening?'—stuff like that . . . She wouldn't answer . . . don't talk to nobody. And if she does, it's snappy—'Mind your own business,' or something like that."

"What is she doing?"

"No . . . can't see what anybody is doing."

"Watch. Concentrate," said an agent. "She's on your right-hand side. You're looking at your arm. Visualize on your screen. You see the small Filipino nurse standing there. Is she touching you?"

"Sh-sh-she thinks she takes care of everything," Neely stutters. "She checks everything."

"What do you see now?" Dr. Spiegel interjected. "What is she doing in this frame?"

"She, sh- stands right . . . right between your head and your belly and looks right down at you."

"Is she checking something? Do you see her hands?"

"Yeah, yeah. She's just doing . . . taking care of everything. You know . . . But I don't know. Maybe she wasn't even there that night. But, uh, I think she was."

"Had you seen her before that night?" asked an agent.

"Yeah . . . In my room. Uh, they both, they both were my nurses, uh, a couple of times . . . in 462, they were my nurses."

Neely's statements are confusing. It does not appear that the suspects were ever his official nurses. Did he mean the two Orientals had visited him before? More questions and answers, however, revealed that Neely saw only one Filipino in his room at the time of the attack—"the one who isn't friendly, the one I don't like.

I shouldn't say that. The one I just didn't get very well acquainted with."

"Now go back to the screen," said an agent. "Clear it ... What do you see?"

"She's got two strikes against her already," said Neely, "and if I say anything more about her, boy, she's gonna have it rough."

"Show us. Tell us."

"Well, it's dark. Well, not that dark, not with the door open and the hall light on ..."

"What do you see?"

"Her and that colored fellow."

"Pancho and Nancy have left. Right?"

"Yes. Left."

"Just before your breathing difficulty?"

"Yeah. Had to be ..."

"Dick," said an agent, "if you saw the Filipino again would you recognize her?"

"Ah, I believe, I believe I most sure would know her."

"You remember her clearly?"

"Yes."

"Visualize her ... You have a clear picture?"

"I don't believe she had glasses on. Can't tell about her teeth."

"Look at her nose. Anything unusual about her nose?"

"There is something," said Neely. "Now ... I wouldn't say that it's her nose ... Mouth? ... Eye? ... What is it? ... But there was something. What the heck was that? I can't, I can't remember that now."

"What do you see, Dick?" asked Spiegel. "Take your time."

"All I see is her running like hell."

"Okay," said an agent. "Stop that one right there. You see her running."

209

"But it looks like she's running out through trees, a clump of trees or a grove of trees, or something like that."

Neely's prior limited recollections of the arrest included believing himself out in a grove of trees.

"Is she running away from you?" said an agent.

"Yeah, yeah," responded Neely.

"Now in the next slide—the next slide," asked the agent. "How do you see yourself when you see her running?"

Neely then responded that he saw a man running "out"—a man "in a black suit" with "a long white coat over it, maybe." Then he saw the man walking "back and forth" at the foot of his bed, and "the girl running out" a window and into some woods. "She got the hell out of there ... Seems like it was light when they were both in my room ... The girl might be running out of the room ... The fella wasn't in such a big hurry ... He was a black man, a Negro ... Occasionally he would walk up and down the hallway and I saw him maybe on the elevator or something like that. He acted like, like kind of a big shit. I was kind of scared of him."

The black man's hair was combed "straight back, as flat as a colored guy's hair could be," said Neely. But the apparent fusion of images into a kind of surreal nightmare seemed to have strained everybody. It was decided to end the second session.

As Spiegel brought Neely out of the trance, the sparsely haired subject's head suddenly swished sharply from side to side, his eyes searching intently.

"You thought for a moment they were still here [the black and the nurse]?" asked Spiegel.

"Yeah," said Neely, apparently startled to have suddenly returned to another time and place. "Was I sleeping?"

The interrogation appears to have yielded only confusion. There was no question that Neely had seen something threatening in his room, but exactly what was still open to speculation.

But whatever it was, it had been very real to Neely.

On the following day, presumably after others had been hypnotized, the investigators entranced Neely for a third time. As usual, the agents did most of the questioning. Spiegel would later say they were "highly skilled ... very commendable in the job they did." Apparently he was there mostly as an overseer, to question only when he felt it was needed. And this was probably as it should have been, for the agents knew the most about the case.

Quickly they brought Neely back to where they had left off the last time.

"Okay, Dick, now remember what you told us about yesterday—the two individuals in your room after Nancy and Pancho left? One was a nurse. Small. Can you see her?"

"Yeah. In my mind, I got her."

"Describe her."

"All I can see is her back."

"What does she look like?"

"Nice. A nice ass too."

"Okay, Dick, but what else? What color hair?"

"Black."

"Is it long or short?"

"Long."

Narciso wore her hair short; Perez, long.

"Is she tall or is she short?"

"Short."

Perez is the shorter of the two, about 5′2″.

"How far down her back does her hair go if you can see her back?"

"Well, she's got it wound up."

"How wound up? A braid? A pigtail? A ponytail?"

"Might be a ponytail?"

"Ponytail?" said an agent.

Another agent broke in: "Is the other person in the room too. Can you see it on your screen?"

"No."

"Yesterday you said there was another individual with her. They were scuffling out the door. Can you picture that on your screen?"

"Tell us what you see," said another agent. "Do you see one image or two images?"

"One."

Spiegel: "Now, Dick, you have on your screen one image and you're looking at her back. Is she going away?"

"Standing alone."

"Are you calling her?" asked an agent. "Are you saying anything?"

"Not very much."

"At this point are you shaking your bed?"

"No."

"How do you see yourself at this point?"

"Sitting on the bed, looking at her."

"How do you feel on your screen?"

"Disgusted."

"Why?"

But he didn't explain it. Instead he started talking about whether the figure had a "yellow dress or a white one . . . I think she had a yellow dress, but I don't know." They brought him back to the room.

"Are the lights on?" asked an agent.

"No. Pretty dark in there."

"She facing you?"

"No, she don't face me."

"Is she the girl you call doll?"

"No."

"Tell us how she stands."

"With her back turned."

"Is she walking?"

"No."

"What is she doing, Dick?"

"Looking down at her hands, or her feet."

"Can you see her hands?"

"No . . . they are in front of her."

"Move the film backward, Dick."

He had trouble.

"Dick," said Spiegel, "move the film backward. You can move it if you choose to. Try describing to us what you're seeing now as you're describing it to us, it will start to move. Go ahead, Dick . . . What are you seeing right now?"

"Somebody's standing there in the room. Somebody's in there."

"What's that somebody like?"

"One of the little dolls," said Neely.

Spiegel: "Tall? Short? Fat?"

"No. Short and skinny."

Taller, Narciso is presumably heavier than Perez, but Perez is often described as having a shapely figure.

Spiegel: "Short and skinny. Okay. Go ahead from there and describe what else you see . . . Just look around on the screen and tell us what you see and then, as you're telling us, the movement will start up."

There was a short pause. Then Neely said, "I see . . . I see the bed."

Spiegel: "Go ahead."

"I see her standing down there by the foot end of the bed."

Spiegel: "Which way is she facing?"

"She's looking the same way I am. She's out a little from the bed . . . about two feet."

"Is she moving or standing still?"

"Standing still."

"You're sure it's a she and not a he?"

"No. That's her."

"That's her. Okay, now what is happening?"

"It shows me sitting on the bed ... I'm looking at her." (Pause.)

"Go ahead, what next?" said the doctor.

"I don't know next."

"Anyone else with her?" interjected an agent.

"Not right then. No."

"See any other movement in the room?" continued the agent. "Looking to your right and to your left. Any other movement?"

"Seems like ... seems like somebody else is there ... but I ..." (Pause.)

"Dick, on your screen," said another agent, "focus very carefully ... Is there anything being done by this person that upsets you? Look carefully."

"No, uh, not, no, I don't think so. She's efficient in everything. Supposed to be good. She thinks so too."

"Dick, you mentioned before that there seems to be someone else there," said the first agent. "Could you tell us what this individual appears to look like?"

"Can you see someone else?" said another.

"No, no. I don't see nobody. But I know there's someone there."

"Well, how do you know there's someone there?"

"I think she talked to him."

"What does she say?"

"I don't know."

"Can you hear?"

"No, not ..."

"Then turn up the volume, Dick. You can do it."

"Is she talking to you now?"

"No. She don't, she don't talk very much."

"How do you know there's another person there?"

"You hear 'em talk or you hear 'em walk."

"Okay," said an agent, "go to when you are shaking the bed."

He does.

"Is the person we were talking about before—is that person still in the picture?"

"Yes. I think she is. Uh, she's there. But I wanted Nancy to come back . . . Nancy and Pancho had left."

"Who came in after they left?"

No answer.

"Okay, let's go back to shaking the bed," said an agent. "Got it vividly?"

"Yeah."

"Okay . . . is that person still standing there? The small one?"

"Uh, no. Not right there by the bed."

"Okay, where do you see her?"

"I don't. I don't see her."

"Can you come back to a picture when you saw her leaving?"

"No, don't . . ."

"What was it that made you annoyed at that time?"

"When I couldn't get my breath and I hollered for Nancy."

"What did you think at that time?"

"I hollered . . . I wanted a nurse . . . I wanted Nancy."

"Did you see somebody in your room at that time?"

"Uh, somebody. But it wasn't Nancy."

"You know who that was?"

"I don't know who they were."

"How many are there, Dick? . . . One? . . . Two? . . . Three?"

"I thought it was two."

"Two. Dick, at this time you have the capability to

divide your screen into two separate screens. What we want you to do is to focus one of these individuals on one screen and the second on the other. Can you do that? . . . Tell me when you see the two."

"I got me in my bed," said Neely.

"Okay, you in your bed. But you see those two . . . What I want you to do is separate them . . . One screen will have the nurse . . . The other the other individual . . . Okay? . . . Now can you see the nurse?"

"Yeah. Yeah," said Neely.

"Is she white or black?"

"Nancy's . . . Nancy's white."

He went back to seeing Nancy sometime previous to his arrest. But then he said, "She and Pancho left . . . She's not the one who ran out. She and Pancho left before that."

"Okay," said an agent, "who was it that ran out?"

"I don't know."

"Man or a woman?"

"I think a woman. Maybe someone else."

"Recognize her?"

"Not like Nancy. I recognize Nancy."

"But do you recognize *this* woman?"

"Yeah, she was, uh, nurse at the hospital, I think."

"Ever seen her before?"

"Yeah, She was my nurse. She was my nurse for some time."

"When was she your nurse?"

"In that same room. If that's who it is, I had a nurse just like her."

"Can you see her in that room another time? Move the film forward or backward," said an agent. "Can you see her in that room now—not the night you shook the railings. But another day or night. Can you see her?"

"No, she had her back turned to me."

"I'm not talking about the night you shook the railings... another time... Can you see her?"

"Uh, no... I..."

"You can move it forward or backward," prompted Spiegel.

"All I see is Nancy," answered Neely.

Getting nowhere, the agents switched it back to when he saw Nancy and Pancho leave the room.

"Okay. Once they left, were you awake the entire time?"

"Yeah."

"Until you had to shake the railings?"

"Yeah."

"Okay. The light is off, but it was on in the hallway. Right?"

"Yeah."

"Now from the time they left until the time you had to shake the railing, how much time elapsed?"

"I didn't think they was up to the desk yet."

This appears to have been a distortion. According to Nancy and Pancho, they had had time to turn away from the front desk—thus allowing anyone to slip by the nurse's station unnoticed—and fix some coffee before they heard Neely. Perhaps four minutes.

"So almost as soon as they left, you had to shake the railings?"

"Seems like I did."

"Okay. Did anybody come into the room after they left in that short period of time? It was only a little while and you were still awake. You must have seen them. Did you see anybody come in? Nancy and Pancho were hardly up the hall. Now picture them leaving and the next thing you know you're shaking the railings. It's on the screen. You just have to tell us. We can't see the screen, Dick. You have to tell us."

"Don't seem like nobody came in."

217

They tried again.

"Now clear the screen, Dick."

"Yeah."

"Okay, is it clear? . . . Now let me ask you this. Who was it at the time that we're talking about in the hospital that you were most fearful of? See if you can put that picture on the screen."

"Uh, yeah."

"Is it nice and in focus now?"

"Yeah."

"Tell us what you're seeing."

"The colored man with the white coat on."

"Describe him."

"Not too tall," said Neely. "Kinda stocky. And he don't talk."

"Where are you seeing him?"

"Right there on the screen."

"Where's he standing on the screen?"

"Right at the head of my bed."

"Is he doing anything?"

"Yeah."

"Tell us what he's doing."

"Looking at the big jug of medicine [presumably connected to his IV lines]."

Spiegel: "All right, Dick, now you can clear your screen. And I'm going to count backwards from three to one . . . At one, let your eyes open slowly . . ."

The session ended.

Why the questioners were not interested in learning any more about the black man is not known. (Perhaps they knew something pertinent that has not yet come out.) But it's guessed that because Neely had earlier told them the black wasn't there at the time of his arrest (which is seemingly contradicted in his trance testimony) the agents just weren't interested.

The session was the last with Neely. What the prosecutors learned is debatable. It seems clear that Neely, at least while hypnotized, recalled a nurse at his bedside in the seconds when he became ill. He also could have recalled a black man. In addition, it appears that his assailant or assailants might have rushed out when he began to call for help. But although at least one of the figures appears to have been a Filipino woman—and one resembling Perez—such a trance-induced assumption might be a mistake. And certainly that assumption, if not hypnotism itself, would not be admissible in court.

They would need fact, not assumptions, for a trial.

But the experts had advised that hypnotism, when properly used, can be a legally accepted method of enhancing memory. And if, in the days to follow, this happened—that is, Neely began to recall the frightening events of his arrest without hypnosis—then his testimony on a witness stand, with defense lawyers able to cross-examine, probably would be admissible. And if he then could identify his assailant, that would be hard evidence. The prosecutors could only hope that this would become the case.

But even though the sessions had not been conclusive, the investigators, it appears, still regarded the experiment a success. For despite the legal and factual uncertainties, it seems they regarded the Neely sessions as providing the first, at least in their minds, solid evidence that Perez had been more than a material witness—that she had been actively involved.

Chapter 18

In January, barely a month after the hypnotic sessions, the prosecution's hoped-for developments began to materialize. Agents checking with Neely reported that he now claimed he could identify the nurse in his room at the time of his attack without the aid of a trance. In fact, he said, his mind was now clearer about many of the details.

For instance, he said he now realized he had made a mistake about the number of people in his room. The "scuffling" had confused him. He was now sure there was only one person who had run out of the room— the little Filipino.

Moving as quickly as possible, the agents took a set of photos to Neely's residence in Osceola, Indiana, a small town near the Michigan-Indiana border. Included in the photos were pictures of Perez, Narciso and a third Filipino nurse. Neely stopped the agent, Daniel R. Russo, one of those who had interrogated him during the hypnotic sessions, as soon as Perez's picture came up.

In a taped interview just a few days following Russo's visit, Neely recalled the identification: "They gave me a bunch of pictures, and the third I came to was her. [Russo] said, 'Now are you sure that's her? Are you positive that is her?' And I said yes. And he says, would I sign the back. And he turned it over and there were about fifteen to twenty names on the back. And I signed my name too."

Apparently others had identified Perez (for whatever reasons) as well.

Back in early November, a U.S. grand jury had begun hearing evidence in the case. Narciso and Perez had been the first two witnesses to testify. On a cold, snowy Thursday they had traveled together with their lawyer, O'Brien, and Perez's three-year-old son, Christopher, to downtown Detroit and spent the entire day in front of the federal panel. Narciso had been excused from work at the VA, where, since shortly after the investigation had started, she had been detailed to correcting nursing papers in the hospital's non-patient educational section.

Perez, it appears, had already quit working at the Ann Arbor VA. Before the investigation started, according to O'Brien, she had put in for a transfer to the Lakeside VA, Chicago, where she was to report in late November. When the investigation had begun to narrow in on her and Narciso, efforts had been made to block the transfer, according to O'Brien. But those efforts eventually had ceased.

Perez and her husband, another Filipino immigrant, had been married in Chicago in 1972. They both had friends in the Midwestern capital, and had met there. Like Narciso, Perez had, in 1971, come to America from Luzon, the largest island in the Philippines, and had been granted her U.S. nursing license in 1972. But that had been in Evanston, Illinois—not Alabama, where Narciso had applied. And born June 29, 1944, she, at thirty-one, although smaller and seemingly younger-looking, was nearly two years older than Narciso. Her maiden name, according to Michigan nursing records, was Leonora Castillo Magabo.

Shortly after becoming pregnant in 1972, Perez and her husband had moved to Ann Arbor and she had taken a job, as Narciso had, at the University of Michigan hospital. But the two nurses, it appears, did not meet until April 1975, just a few months before the mysterious arrests began, when she quit the university hospital and became an ICU nurse at the VA.

According to the Detroit *Free Press*, the petite Asian told friends that she'd switched jobs because "she wanted more contact with patients and more of a challenge." (Also, however, according to the *Free Press*, she later told the same friends that her work at the VA hospital was hard because the institution was understaffed"—the complaint investigators eventually came to look upon as a possible motive for the crimes.)

Although she doesn't receive the almost reverent compliments some of Narciso's friends give, she too is respected by fellow nurses for her professional competence and dedication. One former Ann Arbor neighbor told the newspaper: "It seems to me that you need one of two things to do something like [murdering helpless patients]— a motive or a sick mind. She has neither in my opinion."

Nurses working with the two girls point to their performance August 12—the night eight arrests kept practically every staffer in the hospital running from bed to bed—as evidence of their innocence.

"Nobody ate [all night]," Kirk Cheyfitz quoted one of the nurses as saying. "And Leonie just passed out. And then P.I. got so worked up over the sixth [code] coming and Leonie folding up that she started to get weak in the knees and faint, and then ... she got sick to her stomach."

223

But prosecutors, of course, could interpret the breakdowns in an entirely different, and darker, way.

Perez was in the jury chamber for several hours that November morning. Narciso entered after the midday lunch recess. The jury's deliberations are secret, but the Ypsilanti *Press* reported that O'Brien said its questions dealt generally with "the arrests the nurses attended, their duties in the ICU, patients who received Pavulon, who gave the Pavulon, and under what circumstances."

Where the arrest-causing Pavulon came from has not yet been publicly revealed—if, indeed, the answer to that question is even known. But no one has ever disputed that the Ann Arbor VA's system of handling drugs made it easy for anyone with access to drugs to get the muscle relaxer.

Unlike most private hospitals, the Ann Arbor VA used a drug-dispensing system called "ward-stock." Under this system non-narcotic but potentially dangerous drugs, such as pancuronium bromide, were kept in unlocked cabinets on each floor. The killer could easily have stolen some.

O'Brien emerged from the downtown sessions expressing confidence that his clients were not going to be indicted. "If the U. S. Attorney's office had enough evidence," he told reporters, "they would have charged somebody long ago." He said Delonis was just "fishing" by making his clients appear.

Narciso was ordered to return to the jury two weeks later and spent four more hours answering its questions. When she came out, according to the Detroit *News*, she was both relaxed and occasionally smiling.

"I felt fine inside," she was quoted as saying. "They are very businesslike most of the time . . . I really can't tell whether any of my information helped them. I don't feel they treated me like a suspect."

Pressed for deeper feelings, she said: "I want to get back to patient care. The VA has been a big part of my life, but my plans after this is over are still up in the air. I wouldn't consider going anywhere else until this is all cleared up."

The statements sounded confident, if not optimistic. But according to her lawyer and friends, she had actually been in deep depression.

"It's really pathetic what has happened to her," Caroline Coxe, a nursing floor supervisor at the VA, told the Ypsilanti *Press*. "Some days she would just break down and cry. She sent us a postcard from Mackinac Island where she went on vacation and she was really down."

Kirk Cheyfitz wrote: "At the height of the interrogations, Miss Narciso fled to her home and shut herself in her bedroom, weeping, for most of the week. A reporter talked to her briefly at that time. In a quivering, frightened voice, she would only repeat, 'I am in a very bad position.'"

At one point, said O'Brien, she had lost twenty-five pounds.

But in the face of such reports, most federal investigators continued privately to maintain she was bluffing.

Perez, too, was said to be distraught. But because she was leaving, said O'Brien, things weren't "quite as bad." But the cloud would follow her even to Chicago. When she arrived, she was placed in a non-patient position. Then, on January 13, the Ann Arbor *News* bannered a story across its front page headlined 2 VA INDICTMENTS TO BE SOUGHT. The text said Narciso and Perez, according to reliable sources, would be arrested by February 1.

The story was wrong—at least about the date. But wire services picked it up, and not only did Chicago news media, where Perez now lived, play it up big, but so did newspapers and broadcasters in the Philippines. Perez stoically told a reporter: "I laughed about the report. I didn't feel anything at all when I heard it." In Manila, said O'Brien, Narciso's parents had to be reassured with a hasty letter from their daughter after reading the report. If the nurses are innocent, the story was unfortunate.

Two days later (January 15), just about the time that Agent Russo was showing a photo of Perez to Neely, she was back in Detroit making her second appearance before the grand jury—along with four or five other ICU nurses, also subpoenaed (some say because otherwise at least some of them wouldn't have come).

Published reports say Delonis was seen having "huge cartons" brought into the jury room. And speculation was that they contained the video tapes of December's hypnotic sessions. While each of the other nurses spent only half an hour with the twenty-three-member panel, Perez was kept for approximately three and a half hours.

Did prosecutors confront her with the Neely testimony?

"They asked me about some tapes," several newspapers quoted her as saying as she emerged late that afternoon "smiling and seemingly in good spirits." But she declined further comment.

O'Brien was quoted as claiming nothing had happened in the room to alter his conviction that the probe was "still an open investigation."

Large floor-plan diagrams also seen carried into the jury room hinted that the other nurses had probably been asked where they and others had been during certain arrests.

On February 4, Narciso and Perez were served subpoenas ordering them to appear in nurses' uniforms for a lineup to be held at the Westland Police Department February 11. Westland is a suburb approximately halfway between Ann Arbor and Detroit.

Until this subpoena, O'Brien had been relatively cooperative with the grand jury, objecting to its demands, but never formally. Now, however, the defense attorney filed a court motion to quash the subpoenas. They are "unreasonable" and/or "oppressive," he wrote, chiefly because his clients hadn't even been arrested. Their rights were being trampled, he charged, and quoted Supreme Court Justices Fortas, Warren and Douglas in support of his contention.

Reacting to the challenge, Delonis, for the first time in any public record, named Narciso and Perez as the suspects in the case. He did so in response to questions put to him by Judge Ralph M. Freeman, U. S. Court, Eastern District of Michigan, in whose chambers a hearing on the matter was held the day the lineup was scheduled. Judge Freeman ruled in favor of Delonis. The nurses would have to appear.

Sometime late in the afternoon that day, Narciso and Perez set out for Westland. Again, the weather was freezing. Gathered at the police station when they arrived were agents and prosecutors, suspected victims of the attacks, at least one witness to a believed attack and VA staff members who would also view the lineup for possible eyewitness identifications.

In addition to Narciso and Perez, approximately fifteen other women took part in the lineup. Most of them were Orientals—Filipinos and Koreans—and most were VA and former VA nurses, all being paid by the government to pose in the lines. It is not certain, but sometime during the investigation, Narciso and Perez were probably required to be fingerprinted and photographed in nurses' uniforms. It appears they submitted to this as the lineup was forming.

The formal procedure began at approximately 8 P.M. John McCrery, one of the first to view the women, and the patient whose August 15 note, according to numerous witnesses, had implicated Narciso, recalled what happened:

"We were in a waiting room. Each of us went in separately. They brought the girls in, in three different groups—one of six, another of six, and another of five, I believe. One of the groups had all Orientals. The other two were mixed—Caucasian and Oriental. All the Orientals looked similar. We laughed. I said, 'You're trying to mix me up.' " But McCrery said he had no problem spotting the nurse who had given him the August 15 injection. It was Perez, he said. He recognized her "right away."

This, of course, was in direct conflict with what he had been reported to have said earlier. Acknowledging this fact, he nevertheless said he could still see the "large syringe" in Perez's hand. "She didn't say anything to me. She just stuck it in the rubber coupler."

"P.I." could have been around then, he added, but he didn't remember her at that precise time. He did remember seeing her earlier in the ICU, he said. "Maybe she was right beside me and I just didn't know it."

Apparently he was still somewhat confused about what had happened. But he was firm in his belief about who had given him the shot.

A one-way mirror, it has been reported, separated the members of the lineup from their observers. Presumably they were on a stage, in another room. The viewers were not supposed to say who they recognized until they had private conversations with the prosecutors later. (Maybe each lineup participant was given a number.) This silence could have been imposed because O'Brien was nearby, and the prosecution, until legalities required it, did not want to divulge any of its evidence.

McCrery said that besides himself, Dr. Lucy Goodenday, the cardiologist who, according to her own account, saw much of McCrery's arrest, was also at the lineup. She would not confirm or deny this. But if she made any identifications, they probably would be crucial.

McCrery said he was told that if he wanted any of the girls to talk, he could request it. "But I didn't. I was sure."

Another person who appears to have viewed the Westland lineup was Richard Gasmire, son of Charles Gasmire, the over-eighty victim who suffered a suspect arrest in late July. The younger Gasmire is from Houston, Texas. McCrery remembered "someone from Texas" observing the lineup. And February 7, Gasmire said in a telephone interview that he had been subpoenaed to appear before the Detroit grand jury "next week" to testify about what he'd seen the night of his father's arrest.

Gasmire had flown to Ann Arbor soon after his father had entered the VA, he said. The night of the arrest he was inside the ICU at the foot of his father's bed looking at him. Suddenly, he says, with his father dozing, and apparently in stable condition, he just stopped breathing. "I recognized it immediately and shouted out." At that point, he says, "a couple of other people" rushed over and began resuscitation. "I was kicked out."

So did he have any cause to think the arrest out of the ordinary other than that it was unexpected?

"Yes," Gasmire replied. "There's one fact I'm holding back, and I don't think I should say anything about it until after I've been to the grand jury."

"Well, is that fact that someone walked up and gave a shot into his IV before the arrest?"

"No."

"Well, can't you give some hint as to what it is? There are so many puzzles in this case."

"The only thing I'm holding back is the fact that I noticed there was a nurse standing there next to the bed. I did not see her administer anything. I could identify that nurse. Okay? And her reaction during that night is a little bit important."

"What kind of reaction?"

He declined to discuss it further. Several months later, however, in a second interview, he confirmed that the nurse he'd seen by his father's bed was Perez. He would not say more.

Other viewers of the lineup are not known. Neely wasn't there, according to later court documents. Loesch, the young Vietnam veteran, could have been, said both the Ypsi *Press* and McCrery. But neither was sure. McCrery also said he remembered Lutz. Perez and Narciso had appeared in different groups, he added.

The Westland lineup didn't end until approximately midnight, said McCrery. The next day newspapers reported that some of the Filipinos who had participated—not Narciso or Perez, they implied—were "resentful" of the way they'd been treated during the procedure. But little more was heard of the complaints.

Delonis, especially, had other things on his mind.

Shortly after his hypnotism, the sixty-one-year old Neely's health had begun to fail markedly. His cancer had not been checked by the earlier VA surgery, and he'd developed additional complications. He'd had to abandon plans to attend the lineup. And the prosecutor had been informed at that time that Neely probably wouldn't live much longer. In effect, Delonis realized, it was very possible Neely might not be around if and when there was a trial.

This would be another major blow to the prosecution's case. Like McCrery with Narciso, Neely was an eyewitness on Perez. And as McCrery's testimony had already been put in doubt, Neely's, at least at this time, appeared to be the strongest evidence against Perez. If he died, what he had said informally would not be admissible. For one thing, it hadn't been subjected to cross-examination—the right of all accused.

The only way that Delonis could be sure of preserving the testimony was in a sworn deposition—that is, an official transcript made under courtroom procedures with O'Brien and possibly his clients present to question the witness.

But here Delonis had a further problem. The two nurses—although they had been suspects for six months now—still, as already pointed out, had not been charged. And according to federal rules of criminal procedure, the prosecution could only take such a deposition when someone had been indicted. (The defense was allowed to use a deposition taken before an indictment, but not the prosecution.)

For a while, it appeared the U. S. Attorney's case might regress to where it had been before the hypnotic sessions with Dr. Spiegel. But Delonis was aware there had been some recent changes in federal procedure. He went to the legal literature. Sure enough, a change instituted just two and a half months earlier (December 1) said that in cases where "exceptional circumstances" existed, the prosecution might be allowed to take a sworn statement in the absence of indictments.

He decided to go to court.

On March 1, he filed a motion arguing that Neely's rapidly deteriorating health (he had lost in excess of fifty pounds since his operation), his important testimony and the fact that he (Delonis) had publicly named the two nurses as suspects in the earlier court proceedings, constituted the "exceptional circumstances."

O'Brien disagreed. The government's request was "an unprecedented attempt to compel individuals to answer for an infamous crime when they hadn't even been charged," he wrote in his response. Numerous times during the investigation his clients' rights had been violated, he said—most recently in the "fingerprinting, posing for photos in nurses' uniforms, and participation in police lineups." Granting of the motion would be the "ultimate" violation.

Delonis produced a sworn affidavit from FBI Agent Russo telling of Neely's statement that he had seen a nurse running from his room and identifying her as Perez. O'Brien said the very idea of "refreshed recollection" was "tainted." And Neely's memory had been "shaped," rather than prompted.

But on March 26, U. S. District Court Judge Philip Pratt issued his decision. Again the two nurses lost. For the first time in history, said the Detroit *Free Press*, "a federal court has allowed a prosecution witness to testify against suspects who have not been charged with any crime." An appeal was denied. The date for the deposition was set for April 22—approximately a month later. It would be held in a federal courtroom in South Bend, Indiana. Neely, his condition worsening, would only have to travel a short distance from home.

Although Delonis had earlier named Narciso and Perez as suspects, the fight over the lineup subpoenas had gone unnoticed by the press. But now that the two nurses had been officially named again as a result of a much more important decision, even the giant publications reacted. Both the New York *Times* and *Time* magazine ran stories identifying the two women by name.

Guilty or not, their notoriety soared.

During the deposition court battle, O'Brien had announced that he had a witness of his own he wanted to take testimony from. Richard Collins, a retired cook from Dexter, Michigan, who suffered from heart disease, had contacted him following all the publicity over Neely, said O'Brien, and volunteered that while he and Neely were patients at the VA in January, Neely had told him a "bearded man" had been the last person in his room the night of his attack—not a nurse. This was at the same time Neely was telling FBI agents that he now clearly remembered it was Perez, O'Brien pointed out.

Ironically (and unfortunately) Collins, like Neely, had been told he hadn't long to live, and on March 13, O'Brien went back to U. S. District Court with his own motion to take sworn testimony from a dying patient.

But several days after O'Brien had filed, Collins' medical situation changed drastically. Instead of having only a few months left, said O'Brien, Collins' VA doctors were telling him that if he had an open-heart operation in San Francisco he just might be able to buy lots more time—but he had to hurry.

The sudden change in Collins' prognosis caused O'Brien to wonder if someone wasn't tampering with his defense move, he said. But in the absence of evidence to that effect, his immediate concern became the possibility of memory loss that Collins might suffer. Like McCrery, Collins, if he underwent open-heart surgery, would be put on the "heart-lung" machine. And by this time O'Brien was fully aware of the psychological complications that might result from *that* procedure.

Rushing back to the court, he made an appeal for an

emergency hearing on his motion. Meanwhile, Collins had been ambulanced to the VA and reportedly was experiencing "irregular heartbeats" and "chest pains," according to the Ypsilanti *Press*. Almost at the moment O'Brien was making his appeal, VA doctors announced that Collins had decided from his ICU bed that he didn't want to make any formal statements and they were flying him immediately to San Francisco. O'Brien, reluctantly conceding there was little more he could do, dropped his appeal.

The next day, April 19, with Collins already in San Francisco and preparing for his operation, the Ypsi *Press* reported that two staff members at the VA claimed Collins was "railroaded" into leaving. The staff members were unnamed, but the implication was that hospital officials, wanting a quick end to the murder probe, had "talked" Collins out of Michigan so the prosecution of Narciso and Perez could continue unimpeded.

From the beginning of the probe such charges had simmered just below the surface as low-level VA staffers, such as the shift nurses, reportedly found themselves at odds with their higher-level bosses. But the Collins "episode" appears to have been nothing more than another bizarre twist in a continually mystifying investigation. For April 20 (the very next day), the Ypsi *Press* reached Collins in his San Francisco hospital room and quoted him as saying he had left Ann Arbor of his own volition and fully intended to make a statement to O'Brien when he returned. But in view of Collins' serious surgery, O'Brien could only hope that he *would* return, and that his recollections then would be intact.

During all of this, two bomb threats were received by the Ann Arbor VA. On March 17 and 18, according to the Ypsi *Press*, a "woman caller" notified authorities that there was a bomb planted and set to go off. Each morning, however, searchers found nothing. There had been rumors of earlier bomb threats, but hospital spokesmen denied the reports. Even without the threats, a succession of weird events had kept the hospital, which was trying to get back to normal, on edge since August.

By mid-November, there had been three suicides at the VA since August 12—one a month. Normally, even one a year was unusual. In late August, a mysterious "blue substance" had been discovered in the respirator of a suspected Pavulon victim. Officials investigated it vigorously, only to learn it was harmless cleaning fluid.

Not so harmless was a seemingly unrelated (to the Pavulon crimes, that is) attack on a terminal cancer patient in late September. The man was in the supposedly heavily guarded ICU, but someone was still able to disconnect his respirator and almost kill him. He died soon after, in any case. And with the press mocking the "tight security" the administration had professed to have instituted since the muscle-relaxer attacks, agents questioned a member of the cancer patient's family. Charges were never filed, and the impression later reports gave was that authorities thought the incident a feeble attempt at mercy killing.

It seemed that a sinister pall hung over the institution. And many hospital officials said it wouldn't go away until the Pavulon killer or killers were caught.

Less than a week after Collins left, the sworn deposition from Neely was taken. The press was not admitted. In fact, it has been reported that cardboard was taped over the second-floor courtroom's door transom window so no one could see inside. But reporters who waited outside said the proceedings began at approximately 10 A.M. Neely had walked "stiffly and a little unsteadily" into the courtroom, wrote one, "twice placing his hand against the wall for support."

Inside, said participants, Narciso and Perez sat at a table up front. The prosecution led off, examining Neely for maybe an hour and a half. Except for some refinements, he told much the same story he had told during the hypnotisms. But he now had an intriguing new recollection to relate: while being wheeled down to the ICU, following his discovery by resuscitators, he said he distinctly heard someone say, "This is the third one tonight. The cops is sure to come. This is the third one tonight. The cops is bound to come out."

This could have been someone simply expressing suspicion. But it also could have been someone worried over being caught.

Who made the statement—if, indeed, it *was* made—has not been determined. But it opened the door to even more conspirators than were already suspected.

When it came time for Neely to identify the nurse who had been in his room, a witness to the courtroom proceedings recounted: "He was asked, 'Do you see that person?' He said, 'Yes.' He was asked where, and he pointed her out." It was Perez. She was wearing a red jacket over a white turtleneck. He couldn't remember her name, said the witness, so he described her clothes to make the identification positive.

"Let the record reflect that Mr. Neely has pointed to the respondent Perez," said Delonis.

Neely also recognized Narciso, said the witness. But from where or when, it is not known. "Have you ever seen the two together?" he was asked, said the witness. "No," was the reply.

If the prosecution believed Narciso and Perez had

visited Neely together from time to time—as some of his previous statements might have indicated—such testimony, if it has been reported accurately, didn't corroborate that.

Next the defense took over. What O'Brien did or said in regard to Neely's direct statements putting Perez in his room is not known. But the defense lawyer was aware that in the prosecution witness's pre-hypnotic examination (a legal requirement for the hypnotisms), doctors had recorded, "... mental examination of [Neely] reveals a man who admits to memory difficulty. He claims he is forgetful and that his brother and wife complain of his memory."

Apparently emphasizing this problem, O'Brien was able, it is reported, to get Neely to admit he had earlier given conflicting accounts of what had happened in his room—such as the one he supposedly gave to Collins. "He's a confused old man," O'Brien later said of Neely. "I don't know his intentions, and I also don't know how much the FBI has influenced him." Apparently Neely also repeated his hypnosis confusion about the apparel of his attacker, for O'Brien added: "He didn't even know what color uniform the nurse was wearing—white or yellow."

It "was not your model FBI training film testimony," O'Brien concluded about the deposition.

But O'Brien, of course, represents the accused.

The cross-examination lasted approximately an hour and fifty minutes, said the Detroit *Free Press*. The prosecution then took over for another half hour. Later, when asked about Neely's seemingly conflicting statements about who had last been in his room, Delonis said, "He knew from the very beginning who it was. He just didn't want to get anybody in trouble."

The deposition ended at approximately 4:15 P.M. It

had taken all day. As usual, Narciso and Perez emerged smiling from the courtroom, according to reports, and Perez echoed her attorney's sentiments: "He was confused about everything," she said.

Chapter 19

In late May, word began to filter down that the late-September and early-October exhumation tests were finished and that Pavulon had been found.

Delonis refused to confirm the results, but did acknowledge that they were in. "They haven't gone to the grand jury yet," he said, in explaining his "no comment."

In which of the four exhumed bodies the Pavulon was found is not known. But the newspapers wrote that their sources were saying "three of the four." And it could be speculated (in light of the future developments) that the three were Herman, Oulds and Green. Families of the four said they didn't know.

They still hadn't been told anything about the investigation. "It's something that has been on my mind constantly," Bernice Green, widow of Joseph Green, told the Ann Arbor *News*. "I'm very, very confused ... I remember once I asked if I would ever get a report, and they said eventually." But it had never come. A picture accompanying the *News* interview showed the obviously still-mourning Mrs. Green holding a scrapbook of mementos of her late husband.

Delonis further told the media that indictments were not "imminent." But reporters sensed something was about to happen.

The tissue-test results were crucial to the government's case. With them, prosecutors could prove conclusively that murder had been committed. Not one of those known to have been exhumed was supposed to have been given a muscle relaxer. Their respiratory arrests had been surrounded by mysterious circumstances, and no doctor had been able to come up with a valid medical excuse for them.

In addition, more circumstantial evidence appears to have been gathered against the suspects.

For instance, agents had found a witness who, according to investigators, said she had seen Narciso on the fifth floor of the hospital August 15 near a patient just before he'd had an arrest.

Shortly after the three rapidly developing ICU arrests that afternoon, Dr. Bishop had gone upstairs to the fifth floor and found several young doctors working on a fourth arrest, apparently a man named Russell Fletcher. Leaving that resuscitation, he'd discovered the body of Joseph C. Brown, an eighty-three-year-old terminal patient, also determined to have been the victim of an arrest. At first, both arrests had been accredited to natural causes, but investigators had later changed their minds.

It was near these two patients (Fletcher and Brown) that Narciso had been seen. Supposedly she was in a hallway close to one of the victims, one that would not ordinarily have been used for her rounds. There was no reason for her to have been in that part of the hospital, said investigators. Except to add that the two fifth floor arrests occurred shortly after Narciso had been seen in the area, the investigators would not be more specific.

The evidence again, however, was circumstantial. And, of course, Narciso may have a legitimate excuse for having been there, if, indeed, she really had been there at all.

When asked about the accusation, O'Brien said he'd heard nothing about it.

The news media, too, does not appear to have been aware of the accusation. What they were aware of, however, was that the exhumation tests were crucial.

On June 8, the grand jury investigating the case convened again, and immediately the media began speculating this might be its last consideration of the case.

"Sources close to the investigation believe this week's grand jury session may have been called to fit together the final bits and pieces of evidence before the government prosecutors ask the panel to return indictments," wrote John Barton, formerly of the Ypsilanti *Press*, who, despite the competition between the two papers, had moved to the Ann Arbor *News* at the beginning of 1976. " 'If they haven't got enough to ask for an indictment by this time,' one source shook his head, 'they are never going to get enough.' "

Barton was right—at least in his feelings that things were coming to a head. In addition to the signal provided by the exhumation tests, it was also known that several of the ICU nurses who had earlier testified before the jury were now going before it again. Speculation was that now, perhaps under threats of perjury, they were telling more complete versions of what had happened in the ICU on August 15 and other crucial dates, and that this was also helping the prosecution put everything together.

On June 19, late in the afternoon, the FBI suddenly called a press conference to be held in its downtown

Detroit office. In a terse statement to hastily gathered television and newspaper reporters, Jay Bailey, acting head of the entire Michigan FBI force, announced that at the very moment he spoke, agents were arresting Narciso and Perez on a sixteen-count federal grand jury indictment. He refused to answer any questions after the statement, but the meaning was clear: after ten months of complicated, controversial and perhaps even bungling (for if they were wrong they surely had lost the killer) investigation, the government had finally decided to move.

The two Filipino nurses were charged.

The indictments accused the two nurses of conspiring to "poison" ten patients "with intent to injure," and with the first-degree murder of five others. A conviction on any one of the sixteen counts could result in the Filipinos being sentenced for life, or worse.

The five murder counts included some of the dead victims most obviously attacked: Herman, Oulds and Green from the exhumations; Oelberg, who had only an arthritic hip, and who, along with Oulds and Green, died on August 14, the night it appears the killer roamed and murdered at will; and Brown, the elderly victim discovered by Bishop on August 15.

The ten "poisonings with intent" were the near-fatal arrests suffered by: Lutz in the ICU July 27; Gasmire and Hogan (who had remembered his resuscitators working over him) in the ICU July 29; Richard Neely and Don Cihacz (an unpublicized victim on the same floor as Neely and apparently attacked only minutes later) on July 30; Howard Leslie, the patient suffering only a broken elbow, on August 12; Benny Blaine, John McCrery, William Loesch and Russell Fletcher (apparently the first victim Bishop discovered on the fifth floor) on August 15.

Loesch and McCrery were the only patients specifically identified as having been poisoned with "pancuronium bromide." The reason for this is not clear. But it can be speculated that perhaps only from those two did the government have indisputable evidence that Pavulon had been used.

There were seven "overt acts" cited under Count 1 (the conspiracy count) in the indictment. Overt acts are usually those on which the prosecution believes it has the best evidence, and which it will use as a basis for (hopefully) proving the other alleged counts.

These overt acts are:

—That on July 29, the same day it is alleged in Count 4 that Narciso and Perez tried to "injure" Hogan with a "poison," Narciso gave him a non-depolarizing muscle relaxant. (Hogan died the morning of August 15 from what is believed to have been a natural arrest.)

—That also on July 29, the same day it is alleged in Count 3 that the two nurses tried to poison Gasmire, Perez gave him a non-depolarizer. This was the night that Gasmire's son says he saw Perez standing beside his father's bed.

—That on July 30, Narciso and Perez left the ICU together saying they were going to visit Don Cihacz, the arrest victim whose name had escaped detection. This was the same night that Herman and Neely were poisoned.

—That Narciso "attended" the Code 7 called for Fenton Borst on August 12. This was on the same night as, and right across the hall from, Howard Leslie's code, named in Count 8 as one of those allegedly involving Narciso and Perez. And Dr. Dennis Penner said that while he was frantically working on Borst, one of the nurses out in the hall discovered Leslie. (However, in an October interview, Penner could not name the nurse.)

—That on August 15, Perez entered Benny Blaine's room to give him a non-depolarizer. And on the same day, that (overt act six) Narciso "added an extension tubing to the intravenous line" of patient John McCrery. McCrery's arrest that afternoon followed Blaine's by only a few minutes, and Narciso, at least according to her lawyer, does not deny that she attached the tubing. But she says it was at McCrery's request and only to relieve his discomfort, and that she left him many minutes before his arrest began.

Both women do not deny that they were on duty in the ICU when the rash of codes erupted that afternoon. And Counts 12 and 13 allege that Narciso and Perez poisoned the two men.

—That both Narciso and Perez entered Loesch's room August 15 to give him a non-depolarizer. (Count 14 alleged Loesch's poisoning by the nurses.)

The "overt acts" section of the indictment gave one of the clearest pictures of evidence the government would probably try to present.

At a later press conference, Delonis told the Ypsi *Press* that the trial would probably last "months" because the prosecution "plans to call over one hundred witnesses." Were there surprise bombshells that had eluded outside detection? If so, the case against the nurses would be stronger than appeared.

The indictments again brought the national news media to Michigan. NBC ran two back-to-back reports on its nightly news. The New York *Times* placed the story on page one. It was not long before the charges gave rise to speculation about the motive.

The Detroit *Free Press* said "outrage" over the "shortage of nurses" would be one plank in the government's case. A callous attitude toward death and suffering on the part of the nurses would back up that plank.

The motive wouldn't emerge as "a nice, neat package," the story quoted a source. Rather, it would show itself in a "complex set of factors," including those mentioned.

An unexpected part of the indictment—at least to the press—was a phrase in Count 1 alleging that Narciso and Perez had conspired in the crimes with "diverse other persons to the grand jury unknown." While such "catch-all" phrases are frequently used in indictments to cover all possibilities, its inclusion this time, Delonis told reporters, was because there very well might have been other accomplices.

Given the number of attacks in the mass slayings, it seems logical that others could have been in on the poisonings. More attackers would have meant less risk for the others. Another possibility the phrase suggested was that friends or colleagues could have known what was going on but simply turned their backs. There was also the dim prospect of a silent figure behind the crimes—someone unseen "pulling the strings."

Other possibilities had already been hinted at by the many leads to suspects that had cropped up during the investigation. The "black man," men with "beards," men in long white coats, the remarks about "the cops is sure to come" Neely claimed to have overheard while being rushed to the ICU—all suggested elusive "persons unknown." In addition, even as agents were acting on the charges, friends of Denise Nichol (the VA nurse who had mysteriously died August 7 as the suspicious arrests had heightened) were steadfastly maintaining that she had been murdered by someone other than Narciso or Perez because of something she knew.

What that "something" was Denise had never revealed, they conceded (although, as mentioned in Chapter 4, they had felt she'd tried to tell them). But they believed that Narciso and Perez were innocent and that someone else had caused the arrests.

Rather than subsiding, the fears the VA nurses had expressed at the height of the investigation had intensified during the last few months.

Around Christmas, they said—and the following has been corroborated by O'Brien—Narciso was followed home by a young "dark-haired and bearded" white man wearing sunglasses in a "light-colored old Chevrolet." The man had run stop signs trying to keep up with her and had followed her so closely that he'd actually rammed her back bumper several times.

Stepping on the gas, Narciso had lost the pursuer before arriving home, the girls said. But approximately two weeks later a neighbor had reported seeing a man of the same description walking around the side of her house and apparently, the neighbor thought, looking in the windows.

This was in daylight.

Around the same time, the nurses said, several of them—those who'd been checking into the VA deaths on their own in an effort to clear Narciso—also began to experience harassment, apparently from the same man.

One of the girls said she was followed home on New Year's Eve by the stranger, and after she'd gone into her apartment he'd stood in the hallway and banged on her locked door for fifteen minutes before exiting just prior to the arrival of the police. He'd not said a word, just pounded on the door, with an expressionless face. (She said she'd watched him through the peephole.)

There also had been obscene phone calls, notes displaying knowledge of the girls' whereabouts and habits, and suspicious break-ins. The man might have been trying to find out what they'd discovered (which wasn't much), the girls said. In ways not fully understood by those to whom they talked, the nurses had tried to link the stranger with a mysterious "couple in their twenties" whom several of them said they had seen "suspiciously" walking around the VA during the early August attacks.

They had also wondered if a certain male employee (mentioned in Chapter 4) had somehow been involved in these frightening incidents—not as the dark-haired peeper, but, perhaps, in cahoots with him. But the police—putting together a composite drawing of the lurking stranger, said the girls—determined that he was a suspected rapist (apparently not connected to the male employee) who specialized in nurses.

The girls' beliefs are highly suppositional, and doubtless somewhat paranoid at this point. But they serve to underline that at least some of the VA staff had not accepted the grand jury's charges against the two Filipinos. And stories about the indictments in the local press indicated that the newspapers, too, had reservations about—if not outright sympathy for—the girls.

TWO ACCUSED VA NURSES CALLED "VERY COMPETENT" bannered the Ypsilanti *Press* several days after the indictments. HER PATIENTS LOVED HER was the title of an Ann Arbor *News* story about Narciso.

But the government held fast.

Instead of sending word of the indictments by court officials, which is sometimes done in criminal cases, agents went directly to the girls and handcuffed them to bring them in. Narciso was arrested at her home; Perez, at the Chicago VA. Sometimes shackled, the two were taken to nearby jails to await arraignment; and in Perez's case, extradition to Michigan. The next day at the bond hearings, Narciso was denied bail, and Perez's was set at $500,000—in effect, the same as

Narciso's, for she had no chance of raising that kind of cash.

Led back to their cells, it appeared that they would stay there until the trial began. Adding to their difficulties, it became known, was the fact that Perez was four months pregnant. She needed special care.

O'Brien went to court to get the bonds reduced. In the meantime, the Philippine Islands had learned of the jailings. Front-page articles in the Philippine press began featuring the nurses. Sentiment grew that the two girls were being treated unfairly—if not framed. In an unprecedented diplomatic move, the Philippine government suddenly delivered formal notes of protest to America through channels in Manila and Washington. At least order "reasonable" bonds, the notes asked, and take off the handcuffs.

A famous Philippine lawyer volunteered his assistance to O'Brien, and the Philippine consulate in Chicago sent a representative to Detroit to look into the situation personally.

Delonis said he wouldn't budge from his contention that the two women were dangerous criminals and therefore should be treated as such. But a new bond hearing was granted, and O'Brien called six character witnesses to the stand.

In a courtroom packed with supporters of the two nurses (mostly Filipinos living in the area), Richard Collins, the dying patient who said he could contradict Neely's testimony, and who was now back from his San Francisco heart surgery, said, "I knew 'P.I.' practically from the day she started. She's just about the finest there is . . . She could come in today and give me an IV if she wanted." Curt Branham, Narciso's landlord, told of how he trusted her with his only son. And a physician and nursing supervisor each swore that both girls had "excellent" character and work records.

Jailers even told the Ann Arbor *News* that, amazingly, the two girls had been washing their eating utensils, and had asked for a sewing machine to mend inmate uniforms. "They just aren't the type of people our staff is normally accustomed to," one was quoted as saying.

Delonis said he believed that if the bonds were lowered the nurses would flee the country. The United States has no binding extradition laws with the Philippines, he said, thus "The temptation would be too great to go to the airport and board a 747 to freedom."

But, O'Brien asked, if the nurses were so intent on fleeing, why hadn't they done so before in the ten-month period they had been suspects? In fact, he said, they have proven records of appearing when and where the government demanded without any other compulsion than a subpoena.

On June 28, Judge Pratt, who had earlier decided the issue of Neely's deposition, lowered both bonds to $75,000. The girls could go free if they could raise 10 per cent of that, $7,500, and adhere to some strict regulations: they would have to surrender their passports, agree not to travel out of the Ann Arbor-Detroit area and report at least once a week to an officer to be named by the court.

By this time, a defense committee of the two nurses' friends had been formed, and within several days the money was raised and they were out. Newspaper and television pictures showed a large, cheering crowd welcoming Narciso and Perez as they stepped outside Detroit's federal building for the first time in half a month without handcuffs.

This time their smiles were easily understood.

There was a party that night in Ypsilanti for the two girls. Not only were they out of jail, but Perez had turned thirty-two while a prisoner.

Almost simultaneous with the nurses' release, the prosecution received a further jolt: John McCrery, one of its key witnesses, died of a heart attack June 28 while mowing the lawn in front of his Coloma, Michigan, home.

"That is something else," Delonis is quoted by the Ann Arbor *News* as saying when he first heard the news of McCrery's death. "If it is true, that is just something else."

It was one more bizarre and saddening twist in the case. They had preserved Neely's testimony. But all they had of McCrery's, presumably, were video tapes of his hypnotism and written statements he'd made to FBI agents and others.

Delonis, other than expressing his sorrow for McCrery's family, wouldn't comment on what effect the death would have on the upcoming trial. McCrery's testimony, because he'd switched after his surgery from identifying Narciso as his assailant to Perez, was already a problem for the prosecution. But because, as one government official put it, McCrery's first identification "made more sense," and because prosecutors could possibly explain the switch by "post-pump psychosis," it is speculated that they had already decided to use McCrery primarily against Narciso. The fact that the indictment said one of the overt acts the government would try to prove was that Narciso changed McCrery's IV tube is evidence of this.

But they could also try to use the two identifications to argue that *both* girls had an active part in McCrery's attack.

Trying to prove all this, however, would now be tougher without McCrery to testify. And what the defense will have to say about McCrery's allegations remains to be seen.

Almost as a fiery exclamation point underscoring the

bizarre nature of everything gone before, a small item in the *Herald-Palladium*, a newspaper near McCrery's home town, reported that the day after McCrery's death, his beautiful Husky dog Polar had been struck by lightning and killed while taking shelter during a storm.

So what had started as only an aberration in a hospital's arrest rate had ended as one of the most baffling crimes in medical history. Whether it will ever be solved depends on the outcome of the upcoming trial. And that outcome is by no means certain. The fact that the case has become almost an international incident indicates that many people believe the killer or killers are still undetected, waiting to resume the deadly injections at the first opportunity.

That the crime was a mass murder is no longer in dispute. No one but the killer can ever say for sure exactly how many persons were attacked and how many died. The computer investigators identified twenty "very suspicious" arrests during July and August, and nine more that were judged "moderately suspicious." That's twenty-nine that could have been attacked in only that short period.

As to deaths, the government believes it can prove five murders. Six of the computer's "most suspicious" arrests died. And there are lists in the possession of Ann Arbor VA physicians with thirteen possible dead victims—that is, patients in both the "most suspicious" and "moderately suspicious" category who have died.

And who is to say that the count wasn't still higher?

Why did the deaths occur?

There's very little chance of stopping a clever psychopath, especially one who, as this one appears to be, is able to use his or her (or their) identity as a member of a trusted profession to gain access. But it appears that the problem should have been recognized before it finally was—at least by August 13, following the disastrous night of August 12. If it had been, a lot of lives could have been saved. Since the investigation, physicians have suggested the institution of a records system that would quickly identify any deviation in normal arrest rates. Perhaps that's what the VA should have had in the first place.

There are still many unanswered questions. Several quickly coming to mind are: What will be the outcome of Neely's and McCrery's testimonies? Who was the nurse Dr. Goodenday saw by McCrery's bedside August 15? Were trusted physicians questioned as doggedly as were the less regarded nurses? And perhaps the most perplexing question of all is: How could anyone have done this? What manner of mind-warp could cause a human being to murder defenseless persons in so ghastly a fashion, regardless of the motive?

It is perhaps enlightening to consider that reason may not have been a factor in the crime. A maniac is not subject to reason, and motive therefore does not spring from facts. One point that has not been openly considered during the investigation at Ann Arbor is that the killer or killers might have more than one personality, and that one of the two (or three, or more) would allow this divorce from reason.

On the outside, he or she would seem normal and friendly. But from somewhere inside, perhaps triggered by a sign, a sound—anything—could emerge a monster, a person devoid of sentiment, and capable of snuffing out human life on an impulse. At night, or in the afternoons, this personality could emerge and, with a poison-filled syringe tucked in a pocket, perhaps influence someone susceptible to join in the death-dealing walk through the unsuspecting hospital corridors.

Who was there to stop the deadly mission? The few

security guards? The greatly undermanned nursing staff? The feeble cries of helpless victims?

Perhaps the government has caught the killer or killers. But perhaps it has not. In that case, when will he, she, or they strike again? And where?

NON-FICTION BESTSELLERS FROM POPULAR LIBRARY

- [ ] A CELEBRATION OF CATS, Jean Burden — #08424 – $1.75
- [ ] BELOVED PROPHET, Ed. V. Hilu — #08308 – $1.95
- [ ] GAMES SINGLES PLAY, A. Wayne & J. Harper — #00209 – $1.25
- [ ] GIBRAN IN PARIS, Yusaf Huwayyik — #08425 – $1.75
- [ ] HARRY TRUMAN SPEAKS HIS MIND, Harry S. Truman — #08415 – $1.50
- [ ] JESUS NOW, M. Martin — #08309 – $1.95
- [ ] KATIE KING: A VOICE FROM BEYOND, Gil Roller — #03100 – $1.50
- [ ] NUDE BEACHES AND RESORTS, Ed. R. Swenson, Jr. — #03071 – $1.50
- [ ] THE OTHER FEMALE IN HIS LIFE, Dodo Laric — #08411 – $1.25
- [ ] REAL LACE, S. Birmingham — #08307 – $1.75
- [ ] THE THREE FACES OF EVE, C. H. Thigpen, M.D. and H. M. Cleckley, M.D. — #08137 – 95c
- [ ] WHEN I DON'T LIKE MYSELF, William Hulme — #00345 – $1.25
- [ ] WOMEN IN PRISON, Kathryn W. Burkhart — #08421 – $1.75
- [ ] WASHINGTON D.C. — PAST & PRESENT THE GUIDE TO THE NATION'S CAPITAL — #08368 – $1.95
- [ ] WHO DESTROYED THE HINDENBURG? A. A. Hoehling — #08347 – $1.75
- [ ] WOMAN'S DOCTOR, Dr. William J. Sweeney III with Barbara Lang Stern — #08271 – $1.75

Buy them at your local bookstore or use this handy coupon for ordering:

Popular Library, P.O. Box 5755, Terre Haute, Indiana 47805 BOB-10

Please send me the books I have checked above. I am enclosing $_____ (please add 35c to cover postage and handling). Send check or money order —no cash or C.O.D.'s please. Orders of 5 books or more postage free.

Mr/Mrs/Miss_____

Address_____

City_____ State/Zip_____

Please allow three weeks for delivery. This offer expires 5/77.

National Bestsellers from Popular Library

☐	THE HOLLOW MOUNTAINS—Oliver B. Patton	$1.95
☐	THE LANDLADY—Constance Rauch	$1.75
☐	NINE MONTHS IN THE LIFE OF AN OLD MAID Judith Rossner	$1.50
☐	THE BEST PEOPLE—Helen Van Slyke	$1.75
☐	THE CAESAR CODE—Johannes M. Simmel	$1.95
☐	THE HEART LISTENS—Helen Van Slyke	$1.75
☐	TO THE PRECIPICE—Judith Rossner	$1.75
☐	THE COVENANT—Paige Mitchell	$1.95
☐	TO KILL A MOCKINGBIRD—Harper Lee	$1.50
☐	COMPANIONS ALONG THE WAY—Ruth Montgomery	$1.75
☐	THE WORLD BOOK OF HOUSE PLANTS—E. McDonald	$1.50
☐	WEBSTER'S NEW WORLD DICTIONARY OF THE AMERICAN LANGUAGE	$1.75
☐	WEBSTER'S NEW WORLD THESAURUS	$1.25
☐	THE LAST CATHOLIC IN AMERICA—J. R. Powers	$1.50
☐	THE HOUSE PLANT ANSWER BOOK—E. McDonald	$1.50
☐	INTRODUCTION TO TERRARIUMS Barbara Joan Grubman	$1.50
☐	A BRIDGE TOO FAR—Cornelius Ryan	$1.95
☐	THE LONGEST DAY—Cornelius Ryan	$1.75
☐	THE LAST BATTLE—Cornelius Ryan	$1.95
☐	FEAR AND LOATHING IN LAS VEGAS Dr. H. S. Thompson	$1.75

Buy them at your local bookstore or use this handy coupon for ordering:

BOB-56

Popular Library, P.O. Box 5755, Terre Haute, Indiana 47805

Please send me the books I have checked above. I am enclosing $ _____
(please add 50c to cover postage and handling). Send check or money order
—no cash or C.O.D.'s please. Orders of 5 books or more postage free.

Mr/Mrs/Miss _____

Address _____

City _____ State/Zip _____

Please allow three weeks for delivery. This offer expires 5/77.

Yours Free

(Just send 25¢ for postage and handling)

Our exciting new catalog of POPULAR LIBRARY titles you can order direct-by-mail

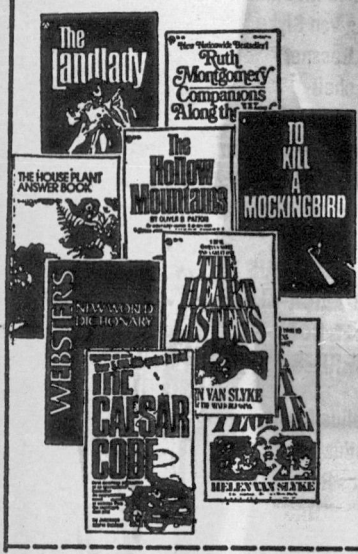

Expand your choice! Stock up on good reading. Round out your collection of books in your special area of interest.

There isn't room on most paperback book racks and shelves to keep and display a supply of all the titles in print.

So we have established a Reader Service Department where we stock all our titles in print and ship them directly to you upon request.

Mail coupon with 25c and we'll send you our latest catalog of Popular Library paperbacks of all kinds: Astrology, Humor, Science Fiction, Sports, Supernatural, Western, Games and Puzzles, Gardening, Gothic Novels, Mystery and Suspense, and much more.

BOB-4

POPULAR LIBRARY PUBLISHERS

Reader Service Department
P.O. Box 5755
Terre Haute, Indiana 47805

Please send me a free copy of your Popular Library catalog of paperback books. I enclose 25c for postage and handling.

Name _____
Address _____
City _____ State _____ Zip _____